Sun and the Skin

Sun and the Skin

Ronald Marks
FRCP, FRCPath

Department of Dermatology
University of Wales College of Medicine
Cardiff, UK

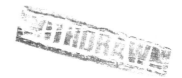
Martin Dunitz

© **Professor Ronald Marks 1988, 1995**

First published in 1988 as *The Sun and Your Skin* by
Macdonald Optima, a division of
Macdonald & Co. (Publishers) Ltd

Second edition 1995
Martin Dunitz Ltd
7–9 Pratt Street
London NW1 0AE

A CIP record for this book is available from the British Library
ISBN 1–85317–275–8

Composition by TecSet Ltd, Wallington, Surrey, United Kingdom
Printed and bound in Spain by Grafos, S.A. Arte sobre papel

Contents

Acknowledgments

I could not have completed this book without the encouragement, help and support of Hilary, my wife. Thanks are also due to my staff and members of the Department of Medical Illustration, University Hospital of Wales.

Introduction

'Bronzed and fit' is the way that most of us would like to be described, but it should be noted that at one time 'pale and interesting' was the preferred description. I am not sure how this change came about, but it is quite plain that a suntan is now regarded by most people as desirable and attractive. However, tanning is only one of the ways in which our skin reacts to the sun. If we stay in the bright sun too long we burn—often a cause for laughter for all but the sufferer. And sunbathing day in, day out over the years causes wrinkling and a variety of unpleasant skin blemishes. So sunbathing has a dangerous side too.

Life depends on the sun. If it were to disappear, so would all living things. If for some reason the earth was drawn a little nearer to the sun we would be in grave danger of being burnt to cinders. The dependence of life itself on solar energy has long been recognized, but it is only comparatively recently that some of the more subtle effects of the sun have been discovered. The effects of the sun on the skin have particular importance, and in this book this aspect of human dependence on the sun is put under the magnifying glass.

Turn the pages of any popular magazine in April, May or June—there is more than a sporting chance that there will be an article, comment or question about suntanning or sunburn. However, alongside the 'fashion' aspects of sun exposure there is a growing tendency to include warnings concerning the hazards of too much sun. We all have more leisure time than previously, and more leisure time inevitably means more sun exposure. Cheaper package holidays have resulted in more people from the chilly, damp and dismal areas of north-west Europe descending on the 'sundrenched beaches' of the Mediterranean, or venturing even further afield. The dose of the sun's energy received in such a two-week holiday in the sun is often considerably more than the average Briton would receive in a whole year at home. But the public are not even content with this 'extra' sun exposure and seem keen to get as much artificial sunshine as possible, succumbing to advertisements for sunbeds, solaria and other forms of simulated sunshine. For these reasons I believe that we can no longer avoid being interested in how the sun affects the skin.

This book is meant for the interested public—for the sun-worshipper and occasional sunbather as well as those fearful of the sun. At a practical level it is designed to answer questions that I have heard time and time again, such as, 'Can I tan without burning?', 'Is it true that too much sun causes skin cancer?', 'Are sunbeds safe to use?' and 'How should sunburn or sweat rash be treated?'

One of our basic human needs is to look good and be attractive. The danger of trying to achieve this in the short term by sunbathing is that, by overdoing it, the very opposite effect is obtained in later years. The various problems that can arise from persistent sun exposure are therefore pointed out. There is also a detailed description of the ways of protecting your skin.

It feels good to be out in the sun, and there is no doubting the psychological boost it gives, especially after a long and dreary winter, but there are other good things about sun exposure that are less obvious. For example, a little sunshine can prevent that unpleasant bone disease in children called rickets. Both natural and artificial ultraviolet light have been used in medical treatments, and to complete the picture I give a description of the various treatments used.

The story of the interaction of human skin with the sun is fascinating at many different levels and it is intended that this book entertains the reader as well as being informative. In places I have gone into some detail concerning the biological mechanisms and the physics involved, in order to satisfy those with a slightly scientific bent. In any case, I think having some background information about the nature of the changes that take place should be helpful.

The effects of the sun on the skin have been enormously influential on our social development and are becoming increasingly important medically. I believe that there is a strong need for information on the topic to be readily available to the public and I hope that this book will both satisfy that need and be enjoyable to read.

1

The sun in social history

A crude disc with 'rays' coming from its edge is one of the first attempts at artistry by infants when given crayons and paper. The appreciation of the presence of a fundamental life force in the sky pervades the entire history of mankind and has infiltrated every aspect of human activity. An awareness that the sun was responsible for warmth and light and was vital to the success of crops must have developed at an early stage in human history, and the movement of this great orange-yellow orb across the sky every day would have been a source of wonder and awe. Its arrival every morning just over the horizon in the east, to banish the frightening darkness of the night and once again supply light and heat, generated myth and religious belief. Imagine the fear and pandemonium amongst our ancestors during an eclipse or a severe black thunderstorm!

All life depends on the sun in a literal sense, and it is scarcely surprising that it became an object of wonder and worship for primitive peoples. Walk around a city in northern Europe at the beginning of summer. Watch the inhabitants with their eyes lightly closed and a look of pleasure on their faces, sitting with their entire bodies turned sunwards. They are celebrating their liberation from the cold, dull, dark and dank days of winter. It doesn't take a great leap of the imagination to see why our unsophisticated ancestors melded the sun into their system of supernatural beliefs.

Sun worship

Sun worship in one form or another has probably existed throughout man's history but we can only be aware of the small number of sun religions that have left some vestige of their culture for us to inspect. Early Egyptian and Greek civilizations seem to have had complex structures with numerous gods and spirits associated with the heavens; for example, in classical Greek mythology Apollo was the sun-god, the charioteer who rode across the heavens daily. The sun-god was often amongst the most important, and at various times *the* most important and powerful, of all the deities. Many royal dynasties have claimed to be descended from sun-gods of various kinds. The Japanese royal family traces its lineage from a great sun-goddess known as Amaterasu; the Emperor of Japan was known as the Sun Emperor, and Japan is still known as the Land of the Rising Sun.

We probably know most about the sun cult of early Egypt. Sun worship in this highly developed culture was centred on Heliopolis, the City of the Sun—now the site of a major new building development in the outskirts of Cairo. The ancient Egyptians believed that the sun-god, Ra, was born each morning from Nutt, the goddess of night. Ra dominated the religious life of the Egyptians, and the pharaohs of the fifth dynasty called themselves 'Sons of Ra'. Their temples to Ra were open to the sky and contained tall stone structures—sun obelisks—around which the religious devotions took place.·

The Incas of Peru and Ecuador and the Olmecs and Aztecs of Mexico and elsewhere in the Central Americas also appear to have had complex systems of religious worship, with the sun as a central and all-powerful god. The Incas of Peru claimed to be the children of the sun. To them the sun was the most important of the sky gods, who were themselves subservient to a Creator God. The stone artefacts that remain from their culture confirm the importance of the sun-god, and their human sacrifices were apparently meant to placate his spirit. The sun has also aided and been the means of religious ritual, even when it is not the highest deity in the particular faith. For example, the Plains Indians of North America, such as the Dakota Indians, gaze at the sun during a protracted, physically testing ritual dance.

In Europe numerous standing stones and monuments remain of mysterious ancient cultures whose religion was probably a form of sun worship. The stone circles of Great Britain and elsewhere in north-west Europe seem to have had great astronomical significance and to have been sites where people gathered for the worship of the sun and the stars. The most famous of these is Stonehenge, near Salisbury in Wiltshire, which has been the subject of a great deal of research directed at understanding both the history and the religious significance of the very striking standing stones. Stonehenge appears to have been used by several cultures, but the fact that one of its central components is accurately orientated to the sunrise of the midsummer sun surely indicates the importance of the sun in some type of religious ritual.

There are other less well-known examples where accurate observation of the sun appeared to be important in the devotional sense. There are burial mounds, containing what are known as 'passage graves', and standing stones in Ireland—at Newgrange, near Boyne, and in the Loughcrew mountains—that appear to date from 3000 to 4000 years BC. The structure in the Loughcrew mountains was found recently to be built to receive the rays of the rising sun at the spring equinox and to make complex patterns of light in the burial chambers within, while at the Newgrange monument the winter solstice sun strikes the end wall of the megalith construction to show the different geometrical patterns carved on the walls.

Skin colour and attitudes

It has been generally assumed that black-skinned people evolved their characteristic skin pigmentation as a protective feature against damage from the sun's rays. Superficially the proposition seems quite reasonable, as for the most part they live in those parts of the world that have the most sun. However, closer examination has thrown considerable doubt on this assumption. The darkest degrees of skin pigmentation are seen in some groups of African peoples who live in the dense rain forests, where hardly any sunlight penetrates at all. Even more challenging to this concept is the fact that, for pigmentation to have survival value for the human race as a whole and thus be of evolutionary significance, it would have to give the more darkly-pigmented people a better chance of having children. However, as pigmentation seems to be important mainly against the development of skin cancer (see Chapter 6), and this develops in later life after the reproductive period, it seems unlikely to have any evolutionary significance on this score. And to make things really difficult, there have been such marked migrations of ethnic groups that it is really quite impossible to know where any one group originated.

Regardless of the biological explanation for the diversity of human skin colour, our social attitudes to skin colour are bizarre and at times incomprehensible. The waggish statement that the world seems to be divided into white people trying to become black and black people attempting to look white is not so very far from the truth. There is no simple explanation for this apparent current dissatisfaction with one's own degree of skin pigmentation. Partly it must be due to the perceived social, sexual and economic benefits of a particular skin colour, although how these perceptions first started is a mystery. However, it seems clear that, once initiated, they are fed and massaged by the media.

Examine the skin colour of a Rubens nude, with the generous folds of skin portrayed in creams and pinks, the lustrous white of the skin of the reclining nude duchess by Goya, the delicate light tones of the facial skin the portraits of the Pre-Raphaelites, the inviting pinky pallor of the salacious, partially-naked girls of Renoir, and the intentionally titillating portraiture of women's skin by any of the classic artists. All are white—or at least considerably paler than any of the men in the pictures. Men's skin is shown perceptibly darker than that of women, and indeed the difference appears to have been a very important sexual 'turn-on' for men.

Poets used to wax lyrical over the fairness of the skin of their objects of devotion. They compared their ladies' complexions to the whiteness of snow, to the feathers of the dove and to the petals of the lily. Paleness of complexion was taken as the mark of gentility in a woman. It was a sign of high social class and a proper feminine attribute. It was preserved by veils, high collars, scarves and broad-brimmed hats. To be ruddy-faced, brown and weather-beaten was identified as a characteristic of peasants and of the lower social orders.

It is not clear when attitudes changed. The turning point may have been in the 1920s when the popular media began to disseminate the image of the monied classes frolicking in the south of France. A cult figure of that era—Coco Chanel—is reputed to have popularized the 'bronzed' look. Presumably 'the tan' then became identified with elegance, grace, privilege, money and leisure. This view gathered pace in pre-World War II years as the idea of the 'right to leisure' grew. Holidays with pay became mandatory in both the UK and France in the 1930s, and about the same time technological improvements in both the means of transport and in communication assisted the trend. In the post-war years the travel boom began. Resorts sprouted where there had been only rocks and dunes before. The development of fuel-efficient jet planes and charter companies that could make a profit on almost 'give-away' air tickets were both an essential component to the 'browning of Europe'.

The travel industry expanded throughout the 1960s and 1970s. Cheap travel became cheaper, and more and more exotic places became accessible to the working population. The destinations certainly varied in the number of temples, museums, shops and sites to see and the type of food on offer, but they all had one major attribute in common—they were places where sunny weather was all but guaranteed. The traditional Mediterranean holiday spots of France and Italy were joined by new resorts in Greece and Spain and, more recently, by those in Turkey, Tunisia and Thailand.

Meanwhile affluence and leisure have grown apace. The working week has gradually diminished and holidays have lengthened. Leisure centres, sporting-goods boutiques and travel agents have mushroomed, responding to the socio-economic needs of the time. For many in the expanding middle classes, two holidays per year has become the norm—the second either a skiing holiday in the winter sun or travel further afield to some hot spot.

So you see how a continuous process of increased leisure coupled with increased opportunity has resulted in increased sun exposure in one way or the other for the majority of the population. Being tanned is now firmly identified with health and with healthy pursuits. To have tanned skin is to show that you have basked in the sun, that you can enjoy the sensuous; it has become synonymous with sexual allure—the very opposite to the attractions of fairness and pallor of a century ago.

This turn-around in our tastes has been massaged and manipulated by the marketeers and media men. An enormous industry is centred around sunbathing and the suntan. Pause for a moment and think of the products that are made specially for this sun-cult—the sunglasses, the sunscreens, the creams to use afterwards, the special clothing, and so on. 'Fly to delicious golden beaches and develop a wonderful golden tan!' say the adverts. And we apparently cannot resist.

Suntan centres and sunbeds

In case we don't receive enough sun exposure from holidays or leisure activities, suntan parlours and solaria have sprung up in suburban high streets, promoting the importance and allure of the bronzed look. Home sunbeds and sun canopies are extensively advertized, with adverts making such claims as 'they prepare you for sunbathing', 'they rectify vitamin deficiencies', 'they are health promoting and "safer than sun".' A survey by *Which?* magazine found that one person in 11 had used solaria, sunbeds, sun canopies or sunlamps in the previous two years. Of these, one in four had used the tanning equipment before going on holiday, and one in nine to keep their tan after they returned. Interestingly, the same survey found that only one in nine people who had bought a lamp in the previous two years used it regularly and

one in five had given up using it altogether.

Spending money on tanning apparatus or on visits to a suntan parlour is at best wasteful and at worst hazardous. Guidelines for the safe use of the equipment by operators of suntan centres have been issued by the government's Health and Safety Executive, but in the survey conducted by *Which?* it was found that, in general, customers were unaware of the official safety guidelines. For example, not all the operators insisted on the correct use of goggles. One reassurance is that members of the Association of Sun Tanning Operators (they display a badge on the premises) have agreed to a code of practice based on guidance by the Health and Safety Executive.

If after reading this book you still feel that you need to be baked a golden brown, at least pay attention to the following. Always wear goggles. Always match the exposure to your skin's reaction. Be extra careful if you are fair-skinned and burn easily. Don't use the apparatus if you have a disorder that is made worse in the sun (check with your GP). Don't wear cosmetics or perfumes before a session. Don't have more than 20–30 sessions per year. Make sure the apparatus is working properly.

2

The sun, sunlight and artificial ultraviolet radiation

What is the nature of the great bright orange-yellow disc-like object up in the sky that we know as the sun and which gives us our heat and light? The answer to this question and others concerning the sun's radiant energy and our attempts at artificially reproducing it are outlined in this chapter.

It is important to realize that the sun is the source of practically all the earth's energy. Indeed, apart from a few radioactive minerals and rocks that may have emanated from sources outside our own solar system, the sun is our only source of energy. All living things derive the energy necessary for life from complex molecules that can ultimately be traced back to green plants and the process of photosynthesis. Only plants have this capacity for making sugars and other molecules by photosynthesis, in which solar energy is

fixed with the help of the green pigment known as chlorophyll. All our natural fuels, including wood and animal fat and the fossil fuels coal, peat, oil and gas, contain energy that was originally obtained from the sun and fixed by photosynthesis.

What form does the sun's energy take and how does it reach us from some 93 million miles away? The answer to both questions is that the energy is transmitted as radiation of different wavelengths across the vacuum of space. The radiation consists of an enormous range of wavelengths. The different wavelengths are known collectively as the electromagnetic spectrum, and this includes X-rays, gamma rays, radio waves, microwave radiation, ultraviolet radiation, visible light and infrared radiation. (Note that I have referred to ultraviolet radiation (UVR) rather than ultraviolet light, by which it is sometimes incorrectly known, as by definition it lies outside the visible light spectrum and therefore cannot be seen.)

The sun

It is the sun's radiation that is our major concern, but before going into any detail it would be useful to remind you of the nature of the sun and the earth's relationship to it. The sun is a star, just like many of the stars that can be seen brightly studding the night sky. It is in the process of burning itself out, but luckily this is not going to happen

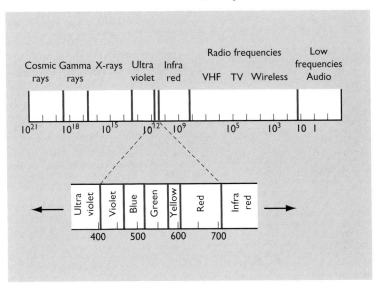

The electromagnetic spectrum. The ultraviolet, visible and infrared parts of the spectrum have been magnified.

for the next few million years or so. The sun is the centre of our solar system and the earth is one of nine planets orbiting around it. However, it is its physical structure that is difficult to grasp. It is hard for the non-astronomer to blandly accept that our familiar and friendly sun is in fact a fiery, globular mass of burning gas with a diameter of 1.39 million kilometres (109 times the diameter of the earth) and a weight approaching 333 000 times as much as that of the earth, stuck some 93 million miles away in the sky. The temperature of the surface of the sun is 5500°C, but its interior is much hotter still.

Although still gaseous, the centre of the sun is also immensely heavy and can be thought of as a sort of giant nuclear generator in which hydrogen is being converted into helium. This 'conversion' involves loss of mass and the liberation of energy as heat and radiation.

The sun's energy is poured out continually and consistently—or is it? In fact there are small fluctuations in the energy it emits, due to sunspots. These appear as darker areas of comparative coolness on the sun's surface. They are of variable size, last for days, weeks or even months, and may recur. At times many spots occur together, and there seems to be an 11-year cycle of sunspot activity. Sunspots seem to represent a type of magnetic disturbance which can be detected on earth and which changes slightly the relative amount of radiation of different wavelengths reaching the earth's surface. Interestingly, the 11-year cycle of sunspot activity can be traced by changes in the growth pattern of vegetation—regular disturbances can be seen, for example, in the annual rings of trees, and these reflect the sun's cycle of activity.

Periods of intense magnetic disturbance also vary within a 27-day cycle—which is the period of the sun's rotation relative to the earth.

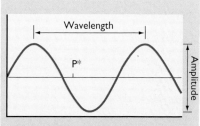

*The frequency of the wave is the number of whole wavelengths passing point P in one second and is measured in Hertz (Hz)

Diagram to illustrate the waveform of the various parts of the electromagnetic spectrum, showing wavelength, amplitude and frequency.

Solar radiation

It used to be thought that light consisted of particles, but this idea was gradually displaced by the wave theory of light. Despite the many advances he made in understanding the behaviour of light and the nature of colour, Newton believed that light was particulate in nature. It wasn't until an English physician, Thomas Young, published the results of his studies at the beginning of the nineteenth century that good evidence was produced for the wave theory of light. We now think of all the radiant energy of the sun being in the form of waves of energy of different wavelengths—the electromagnetic spectrum.

Radiation can be imagined as travelling like a wave on a shaken rope or a ripple in a pond after dropping in a small stone. The wavelength is an important characteristic of any type of radiation and describes the distance travelled by the wave in one complete cycle. Do not confuse this with either the frequency of a radiation, which describes the number of cycles that pass a particular point per second, or the amplitude, which is a measure of the vertical distance of the trough or crest of the wave to the centre line.

Wavelengths in the electromagnetic spectrum are measured in metres. Some radio waves have wavelengths measured in hundreds of metres, but the wavelengths of visible light are

Ultraviolet   Visible light   Infrared

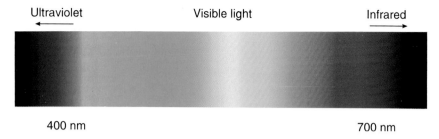

400 nm   700 nm

The visible part of the electromagnetic spectrum showing the boundaries with the ultraviolet and infrared parts.

very much shorter, so short that they are measured in nanometres—a nanometre is a thousand-millionth of a metre, i.e. 10^{-9} metres (0.000 000 001 metres).

Our major interest in this book is in ultraviolet radiation (UVR), because this is the section of the electromagnetic spectrum that has most bearing upon the effects of the sun on the skin. This is the case even though 50 per cent of the sun's energy that reaches the earth's surface is in the visible portion of the spectrum and only 5 per cent is in the UVR part of the spectrum. The ultraviolet section of the solar spectrum is, by convention, itself divided into long, medium and short wavebands—UVA, UVB and UVC respectively. UVB (280–320 nanometres) is biologically the most important part of the ultraviolet seg-

ment, but UVA (320–400 nanometres) is also quite important. The sun's UVC radiation has no biological importance for humankind, simply because none of it actually reaches the earth's surface—it is filtered out by the earth's atmosphere and the ozone layer. The atmosphere is the envelope of gases surrounding the earth and consists mainly of nitrogen and oxygen. However, some 15 to 30 kilometres up into the atmomsphere there is a thin but vitally important layer of ozone gas (a special form of oxygen). Although only about 2.5 centimetres (1 inch) thick on average, the ozone layer allows life to exist on the surface of the planet; without it the amounts of ultraviolet radiation that would reach the earth's surface would kill off most plant life and ultimately all animal life! As an example of the importance of the ozone layer, it is worth mentioning a recent calculation of the effects of reducing its thickness. The researchers who made the calculation said that if the amount of ozone in the atmosphere was reduced by 2 per cent, the rise in UVR would cause an extra 142 000 cases of skin cancer per year in the United States by the year 2025!

The reason for spending a little time on this aspect of solar radiation is that there is a real danger that the ozone layer may be reducing in thickness because of our inability to control the undesirable side-effects of modern technology. The exhausts from high-flying jets have a small but definite destructive effect on the ozone layer, but probably of more importance has been the discharge into the atmosphere of inert-gas propellants from aerosol cans. The chlorofluoromethanes released in this way interact with the ozone and gradually destroy it. It is odd to think that anything so apparently harmless as the fashionable urge to keep our armpits odour free could be quite so threatening to the continued existence of life on the planet! Refrigerants, insulating materials and fire retardant substances may also be destructive to the ozone. Observations suggest that there is a hole in the ozone layer over the Antarctic which is growing. Relative thinning of the ozone layer has also been detected over northwest Europe and there is little doubt that there is a serious threat to the integrity of this protective layer around our planet. Scientists and legislators have joined together to try to stem the loss of ozone. Their combined activities have resulted in the chemical industry voluntarily synthesizing new and less destructive agents so that it is likely that within the next decade the trend to ozone thinning will be slowed or even reversed.

What influences the solar UVR reaching the earth

From the above it is clear that the amount of ozone in the atmosphere and the thickness of the atmosphere has a major effect on the amount of UVR that reaches the earth from the sun. Thus the lower a place is relative to sea level, the less UVB radiation that penetrates. At the Dead Sea in Israel—at 400 metres below sea level, the lowest point on the earth's surface (see page 80)—much of the sunburning UVB is filtered out by the 'extra' amount of air above the earth's surface, allowing relatively more UVA to reach the surface. As a further example you should be reminded of just how easy it is to be seriously sunburnt when mountain climbing. In fact we can expect about a 4 per cent increase in the sunburning effect of the sun's rays for each 300 metres that we climb.

We are all aware of the difference that latitude makes—the nearer the equator, the hotter it becomes. This is primarily a matter of the position of the sun in the sky and the decreased distance that the rays have to travel through the atmosphere. The nearer the equator, the higher the sun is in the sky; the sun's rays therefore approach the earth's surface vertically. Further away from the equator the sun is lower in the sky and the sun's rays approach the earth's surface at an angle, therefore having to travel a greater distance through the earth's atmosphere.

Apart from latitude, however, there are two other factors that influence the amount of UVR at the earth's surface—the season of the year and the time of the day. In the UK something like 130 times the amount of sunburning UVR reaches the skin at noon in mid-June as at noon in midwinter. Interestingly, even though the height of the sun is similar in April and May to that in August and September, the sunburning power of the sun's rays is greater in the late summer months. This is because of slight seasonal changes in the thickness of the ozone layer. Two other factors could possibly explain the increased effectiveness of the sun's rays in August and September—the humidity and wind currents. Experiments by a research group working in Texas have found that both factors can increase the effects of UVR on mice, independently of their effect on the amount of solar infrared radiation that reaches the skin.

The heat energy of the sun is contained mainly in the infrared waveband, and experiments have shown that heating the skin over long periods can cause damage similar to that produced by UVR. It is still quite common to see an odd network pattern of brown discolouration of the skin on the lower legs of elderly people who have warmed themselves repeatedly during the win-

ter in front of a small coal or gas fire. These tell-tale signs of the inadequacy of our domestic heating arrangements can even (although rarely) progress to the point of developing a small skin cancer, just as with chronic exposure to the sun (see Chapter 6).

So far we have dealt with latitude, altitude, season and time of day—the invariable factors that determine the dose of UVR received—as well as some variable climatic factors such as wind, heat and humidity. Other factors that may also alter the amount of solar radiation that reaches the earth's surface include the amount of cloud in the sky, the amount and type of atmospheric pollution, and the concentration of carbon dioxide in the atmosphere. Cloud obviously obstructs the UVR, though by no means completely. It is important to know that even if there is cloud cover it is still possible to get sunburnt in Mediterranean climates and other countries near the equator although in the UK this is very unlikely, if not impossible, even in midsummer. Pollution decreases the UVR reaching the earth because of the light-scattering properties of the suspended particles in the atmosphere, whilst gases will both absorb and diffuse the solar UVR.

The type of environment is also important in calculating how much radiation will reach the skin. Snow-covered surfaces, for example, reflect a great deal of solar UVR—more than any other natural surface. This is why it is so easy to get sunburnt during a skiing holiday and why the eyes tend to become sore and bloodshot if un-protected whilst skiing. Quite a lot of UVR is reflected from sand (depending on how clean and white it is) and some gets reflected by water, although not nearly so much as from snow. Ordinary window glass cuts out all but the longest UVR wavelengths, so that you can't be sunburnt sitting behind a window. However, by alter-ing the chemistry of the glass it is pos-sible to build in any required filter properties needed.

All these climatic and environmental factors have to be taken into account when calculating the amount of UVR received at a particular point—a com-plex task. In fact it is even more com-plex than I have described, because the physics involved is quite difficult and not really completely worked out. However, it may be important to esti-mate how much UVR individuals receive in particular jobs or in various activities in order to provide advice and, where necessary, protection. In recent years this task has been made much easier by the development of personal dose meters or dosimeters. These are badges that contain film made of a special material known as polysulphone. They are worn on the lapel, and they gradually darken according to the amount of UVR that they absorb. They are quite similar in concept to the badges worn by workers who may be exposed to X-rays or radioactivity. There are other devices, known as radiometers, that measure more accurately than the polysulphone badges, but they are less useful for

determining the level of personal expo-sure.

It is interesting to learn of some of the findings that have been made using personal dosimeters. The following fig-ures are the fractions of the dose received compared to the ambient dose that reaches an unshaded horizon-tal surface. Sunbathing on a beach, for example, gives a figure of 0.75, while sitting by a swimming pool gives a fig-ure of 0.40. Skiing results in a fraction of 0.22, and sailing results in a fraction of 0.14, while gardeners receive 0.1 of the available UVR dose. Laboratory and office workers receive only 0.03 of the available UVR, so you can see what a difference a two–week holiday in the Mediterranean and a week's ski-ing trip per year make to the total accu-mulated UVR dose to the average office worker!

Artificial sources of UVR

These are often known as sunray lamps and, although they attempt to mimic the sun's output of UVR, they often fall far short of this objective. Ordinary tungsten light bulbs emit no (or extremely little) UVR. Virtually all the sunlamps in current use employ the principle that when electrons are made to bombard a gas, various kinds of radiation result. Lamps used for treat-ment are mostly long fluorescent tube lamps in which an electric current (i.e. electrons) is passed through mercury gas under low pressure and the inside of the glass tube is coated with a phosphor material to 'boost' the radiation. This type of lamp emits what is known as a line spectrum—only certain wavelengths, mainly in the UVB range, are produced. In some lamps there may also be a considerable amount of UVC emitted, which is unfortunate as the sun's rays reaching the earth contain no UVC.

For various testing purposes it is better to have a lamp which emits ultraviolet radiation rather more similar to solar UVR than the fluorescent tubes just described. Lamps that can emit a more or less continuous spectrum just as the sun does are known as solar simulators—the xenon-arc type of lamp is an example of this kind. These lamps need a high current (e.g. 100 amps) and operate under high pressure. This makes them expensive and considerable skill and care is required in their construction and operation.

It is sometimes necessary to see if patients are sensitive to UVR of particular wavelengths. A special instrument called a monochromator is used for this purpose. This device uses a prism or a diffraction grating to separate the various wavelengths so that with special optical equipment it is possible to shine the test wavelength on a very small area of the patient's skin.

Lamps used for the treatment of psoriasis by PUVA (see pages 78 and 79) are made specially to radiate predominantly in the UVA wavelengths. As the whole body is treated, the lamps are mounted in step-in cabinets or boxes or on hanging canopies over special beds. The lamps used by suntanning parlours are mostly similar to PUVA lamps.

Doctors are often asked whether it is worthwhile buying a sunlamp to use in the home. My own view is that it is hardly ever justified. Even if the individual concerned has a skin disorder that responds to UVR treatment, such as psoriasis or acne (see Chapter 8), it is better to have the UVR administered safely and efficiently by experts and the effects regularly monitored by staff trained in the use of the specialized lamps. Anyway, for the most part the usual lamps on sale are too small and not suitable for proper UVR treatment. Of course there are exceptions. Some patients may not be able to visit the hospital or clinic regularly for the treatment, and may be taught the potential dangers and the various techniques but, in general, home treatment with UVR is not a good idea.

3

Skin and its protective function

For the most part, we take our skin for granted. It is only when something goes wrong with it that we appreciate how important it really is. Its protective role is really important for our health. The outer layers of the skin make us 'leak proof' and prevent us losing water and vital body constituents to the outside world. This is why patients who have been severely burnt become dehydrated and have to be given large amounts of fluids directly into their veins. This waterproofing from the outer layers of the skin works both ways—it also stops us absorbing water when we take a bath or go for a swim.

The same outer layers prevent us from being poisoned when we come into contact with harmful materials in the environment. Actually the skin isn't quite perfect as a protector against poisons, as there are a few poisons that can penetrate the skin and cause problems. We can also absorb some drugs through the skin. For example, in some countries you can now buy plasters that contain a drug (hyoscine) to stop travel

sickness. They are meant to be stuck behind the ear, where the skin is quite thin, so that the hyoscine is gradually absorbed.

Apart from these functions, where the skin behaves as a protective membrane, the skin also acts as a mechanical barrier. Harmful bacteria, fungi and viruses are usually prevented from penetrating the skin because of its barrier quality. Generally it is only when the barrier has been 'breached', as with a cut, graze, scratch or insect bite, that disease-producing microbes can gain a foothold. Skin diseases, too, result in a faulty barrier, so that potentially harmful micro-organisms can invade the body.

Look at your hand as you move your fingers and clench and unclench your fist and watch your skin bend and stretch. Its mobility and elasticity are essential to normal movement. When the skin is abnormal, as in eczema or the common skin disease psoriasis, the skin loses its mobility and elasticity and cracks when movement takes place. These cracks are painful and quite disabling, so that somebody even with only their palms and soles affected by a skin disorder may be quite helpless.

The outer layers of skin also 'insulate' against heat and UVR to some extent but unfortunately are not very efficient at this so that other protective mechanisms are also needed (see Chapter 9).

We think of the skin as soft and delicate, but the outer layers of healthy skin are actually quite tough. I do not advise that the more adventurous readers experiment on themselves, but the skin is not easily penetrated by sharp objects. Of course it depends on the sharpness and force that is used, but everyday 'non-combative' contact with objects in the environment does not usually result in injury.

An important skin function that should be mentioned briefly here is its function in visual communication within the community. The skin bears what are known as the secondary sex characteristics, such as the gender specific hair distribution, which are important in sexual signalling. It is also important in identification as a member of a social group so that normality of skin seems to be important in acceptance within a community.

The outer layers of the skin

All the functions mentioned so far in this chapter are entirely due to the qualities of the outer layer of the skin, known as the stratum corneum or horny layer. Over most of the body the horny layer is very thin—about 0.01–0.02 mm thick—but on the palms and soles it is about 0.5 mm thick. It consists of a series of tough plate-like cellular structures called corneocytes which fit closely together and are stacked up in layers. The corneocytes have a tough outer wall of protein and a system of fibres within them consisting of another important pro-

tein known as keratin. At the skin surface these corneocytes are slowly shed one by one in a process known as desquamation. Despite this shedding the thickness of the horny layer stays the same because new corneocytes are formed below from epidermal cells belonging to the epidermis. In skin diseases like the common scaly skin disorders known as psoriasis and eczema there are difficulties in the formation of the horny layer, and instead of the corneocytes being quietly and invisibly shed one by one they are shed in clusters and chunks which can easily be seen. It is these clusters and chunks that are responsible for the appearance of scaling in these diseases.

It always astonishes me that the stratum corneum accomplishes all its varied protective functions even though it is quite thin and is being perpetually renewed. The process in which the dead horny layer is formed from the living epidermis is quite complex and is known as keratinization. It is this process that is disturbed when the skin visibly peels off in sunburn or becomes scaly in skin disease.

The horny layer renews itself every 12 to 14 days; that is, it takes some 12 to 14 days for a newly-formed corneocyte at the bottom of the horny layer to reach the surface and drop off. To keep up with this process of continual renewal, new epidermal cells (known as keratinocytes) are for ever being formed at the base of the epidermis (in the basal layer). The newly-formed epidermal cells then take about 14 days to move upwards to the bottom

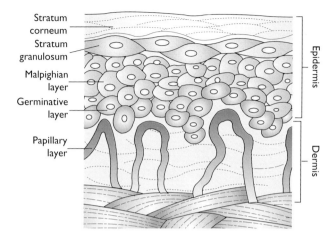

Stratum corneum
Stratum granulosum
Malpighian layer
Germinative layer
Papillary layer

Epidermis

Dermis

Diagram to show the epidermis, the stratum corneum and the top part of the dermis.

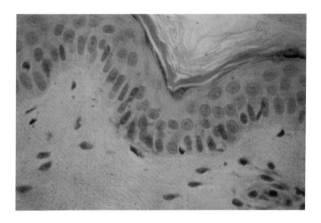

High power photomicrograph to show normal epidermis.

of the horny layer. As they move upwards through the layers of cells above the basal layer (the Malpighian layer) they gradually mature, and this continues in the area just below the stratum corneum where the cells develop irregular granules (the granular layer).

The sun's UVR penetrates the epidermis and affects both new epidermal cell production and the process of keratinization. The kinds of changes produced are described in more detail in Chapters 4, 5 and 6. It is worth mentioning at this point, though, that vitamin D production in the skin is dependent on UVR penetrating epidermal cells to reach a particular chemical compound known as ergosterol. This is important in the prevention of rickets, the once-common bone disease in children, and in the prevention of bone softening in the elderly (see Chapter 5).

In the basal layer of the epidermis there are also special cells which are not of the same type as the ordinary basal epidermal cells. These are the pigment-producing cells—the melanocytes. How they produce pigment in response to sun exposure, and some other details of the skin's protection against UVR, are discussed later in this chapter. Apart from the pigment-producing cells there is one other type of cell within the epidermis that ought to be mentioned. These are the Langerhans cells, named after the Austrian anatomist who first described them in the mid-

dle of the nineteenth century. They have some similarities to the melanocytes, in that they are not true epidermal cells, but they differ from them in that they remain in the middle of the epidermis rather than in the basal layers of the epidermis. The Langerhans cells' main role seems to be in dealing with foreign substances that penetrate the skin, in such a way that an immunological attack is mounted on them. Interestingly, this important immune function has only been recognized in the past 20 years. The Langerhans cells are important to us here because of the way that UVR affects their function, and their possible involvement in the development of skin cancer as a result of perpetual sun exposure.

The microscope section below illustrates the complex ridges and patterns on the surface of the skin of the forearm. These markings, which are exag-

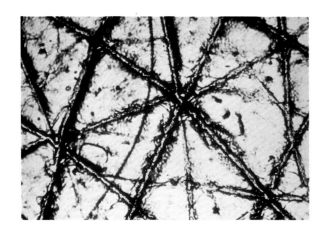

This photograph is of a thin specimen of the stratum corneum from the forearm examined in the horizontal plane.

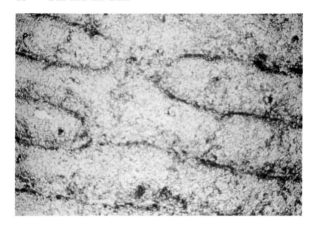

Stratum corneum from the palm examined in the horizontal plane.

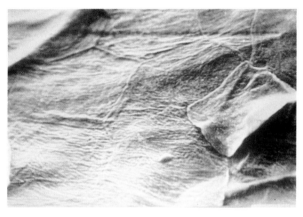

Surface of the skin showing a single horn cell peeling off in the process of desquamation. This photograph was taken using a scanning electron microscope and is magnified about 250 times.

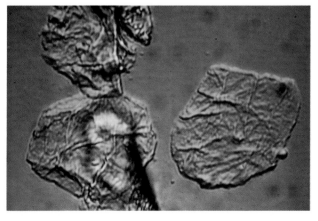

Single horn cells greatly magnified. Note the shield shape and the ridges on the cell surface.

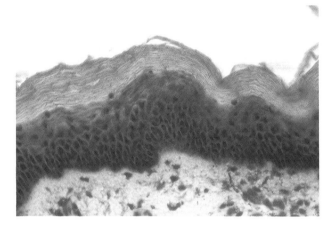

Photomicrograph of skin which has been treated in a special way to show the delicate arrangement of the horn cells in the stratum corneum.

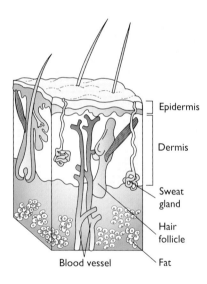

Epidermis

Dermis

Sweat gland

Hair follicle

Blood vessel

Fat

Three-dimensional view of the skin, showing the relationship between the different structures. Note the hairs and their 'roots' (the hair follicles) and the sweat glands.

gerated on the palms and soles to form the well-known fingerprint pattern, are important in allowing the skin surface to stretch and in assisting our grip. The pictures on page 20 demonstrate the complexity of the skin surface. However, we ought not to think of the skin only as a two-dimensional surface. When we consider the way the skin is put together and the way

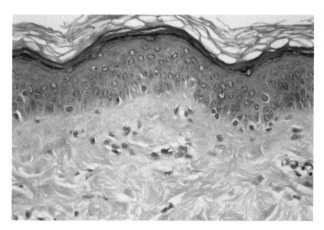

Normal skin showing both epidermis and dermis.

it functions it is useful to think of it more as a three-dimensional structure (see illustrations on pages 21-22). The ridges on the skin surface also partially explain why the epidermis has a 'wavy' pattern.

Hair follicles and sweat glands

The skin surface is studded by two kinds of openings. The first is the hair pore through which the hair shaft pokes. Hairs come from special structures known as hair follicles, which are really part of the epidermis. An example is shown on page 23. It is as though fingers have been stuck into the epidermis to form blind-ending pouches. These epidermal pouches are the hair

follicles, from the bottom of which the hair shafts grow. Attached to the sides of the hair follicles are the oil glands (known as sebaceous glands). The hair follicles vary greatly in size in different parts of the skin, at different times of life and in different ethnic groups. They also differ somewhat between the sexes. The hair follicles over the scalp are obviously very prominent. They are also quite large over the face, but here most of their prominence is due to comparative enlargement of their oil glands. It is these follicles in particular that become involved in acne.

The sweat glands are also epidermal structures but the blind-ending tubes are longer than the hair follicles, and are coiled. There are actually two sorts of sweat gland. One sort is found over most of the body; these are known as the eccrine sweat glands. The other type of gland, known as the apocrine gland, is found only around the genitalia and in the armpits and groin. The apocrine glands don't actually open directly onto the skin surface but drain into large hair follicles. Not a great deal is known about the function of these glands but if they have the same function as similar glands in other mammals it is quite probable that they produce chemical substances (pheromones) having subtle odours that have a sexual role. Their secretion is thick and creamy, in contrast to the watery secretion of the eccrine glands.

In fact the secretion of the eccrine glands is basically a weak salt solution. Large volumes may be secreted in hot weather, when we exercise or when we have a fever. The evaporation of this aqueous fluid helps cool the skin surface and keep the body's temperature down. If we venture into a tropical climate we may secrete very large volumes of sweat until we become acclimatized and secrete smaller volumes after a few weeks. When, as happens rarely, children are born with a deficiency in the eccrine glands, the body temperature can rise dangerously because of the absence of this cooling effect of sweat.

The dermis

So far the top parts of the skin have been described, as well as those structures that open at the skin surface. We

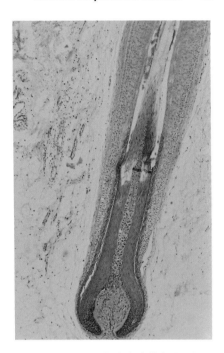

Photomicrograph of a hair follicle. In the centre of the hair follicle there is the hair shaft and at the bottom the hair-producing cells are wrapped around the hair papilla.

must now turn our attention to the parts of the skin below the epidermis, known collectively as the dermis (see illustration on page 22). This structure below the epidermis consists of the fibrous elements of the skin—the component of animal skin that becomes transformed into leather after processing. It also contains the blood vessels and nerves of the skin. It is this deeper part of the skin that binds the softer underlying parts together and gives it its strength. Most of the mechanical strength of the skin comes from the major system of fibres of the dermis—the collagen. Collagen is a special sort of protein that is produced by cells called fibroblasts, scattered throughout the dermis. The fibres are laid down in a mesh, the arrangement of which is far from haphazard and varies according to the particular part of the body. The collagen fibres are interwoven with other fibres known as the elastic fibres, which are also produced by the fibroblasts. Funnily enough, the elasticity of the skin is not due to these elastic fibres but is really due to the extensile properties of the collagen fibre network of the dermis. The elastic fibres seem to have the particular function of binding the collagen network together. The whole dermal fibrous structure is embedded in a jelly-like material called 'ground substance', composed of a group of substances known as proteoglycans.

Tough as it is, the fibrous dermis may be badly damaged by the sun's UVR, especially in the upper part of the dermis just beneath the epidermis. However, the damage caused by the sun takes an odd form. The affected areas of dermis take on some of the biochemical characteristics of elastic tissue rather than the usual collagen. This alteration causes changes in skin texture, mechanical properties and colour. It is known technically as solar elastotic degeneration or more simply as solar elastosis. This type of damage is described in more detail in Chapter 5.

All tissues require a supply of oxygen and nutrients and need some way of disposing of their waste products. These vital functions are the responsibility of the blood and the blood vessels that carry it. The thin epidermis has no blood vessels of its own but manages to receive sufficient of what it needs from the thin-walled capillary blood vessels immediately below the basal layer of the epidermis. These capillaries take the form of loops that poke up in small hillocks of dermis, known as dermal papillae, into the epidermis. The other blood vessels of the skin are lower down in the dermis, forming a series of horizontally-organized networks or plexuses. It is these blood vessels that widen when the skin becomes inflamed and reddened, as in sunburn. The redness is due to two things. Firstly the vessels widen, so that there is more blood in the tissues. Secondly, more oxygen-rich blood floods into the area through the widened blood vessels; this is redder than blood in the veins, which contains less oxygen, so the skin looks pinker. Research indicates that the blood vessels widen in sunburn because of the damage to the epidermal cells caused by the sun's UVR. The damaged epidermis releases particular chemicals that widen the blood vessels and produce all the other signs of inflammation that bother us in sunburn.

A major skin function that I haven't mentioned so far is the one of sensation. Life would be pretty grim without the sense of touch. It would also be fairly dangerous if we had no sense of pain. In fact those unfortunate individuals who are born without sensation may suffer the most dreadful injuries and chronic ulcers, simply because they have no sense of pain to warn them of impending damage. This is also what happens in some kinds of leprosy where the infection damages the nerves to the skin. The various sensations of touch, pain, heat and pressure are detected by special organs just below the epidermis. These are like miniature electronic devices that convert the sensation that they detect into electrical signals which are conducted to the brain or spinal cord by nerve fibres.

Skin colour—why some tan and others don't

'I can't go out in the sun without looking like a lobster', you will hear some fair-skinned friends complain. Others will say that they only seem to tan, and never to burn. What is the reason for this marked difference in the way people react to sun exposure?

Mostly it is due to differences in the amount of protective brown-black melanin pigment present in the skin. In general, the duskier your skin colour the better protected you are against the damaging effect of the sun's rays. This doesn't mean that black-skinned individuals can't get sunburnt—they can! It merely depends on the dose of sun exposure that they experience. In fact our skin colour is the result of many different factors and properties. The two main factors that determine how brown or how pink the skin is are the rate of melanin production and the blood supply to the skin.

I want to discuss the pink colour first. Pinkness (or redness) depends on the red oxygen-carrying pigment in the red blood cells, known as haemoglobin. The greater the rate of blood flow and the nearer to the skin surface the blood vessels, the pinker the skin appears. If we are anaemic or the blood flow to the skin is reduced (as in cold weather), we look pale. If for some reason the blood can't pick up enough oxygen in the lungs, the blood looks somewhat bluish (this is called cyanosis), and that's the colour we look if we are unlucky enough to get pneumonia (it has absolutely nothing to do with royalty or noble birth!). The degree of pinkness, whiteness or blueness doesn't influence whether we tan or burn, because the blood vessels are beneath the delicate epidermis which becomes damaged by the sun.

Brownness of the skin is much more important for protection against the sun. But how does melanin protect against solar damage? The answer is that melanin is black, and black absorbs the sun's rays, whereas white materials tend to reflect all the rays. The amount of melanin that your skin produces depends not only on the amount of stimulation it receives, but also on

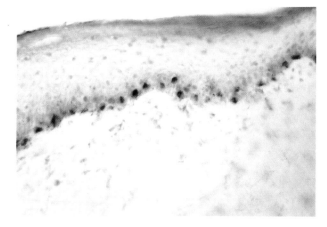

Stained pigment cells (melanocytes) at the base of the epidermis.

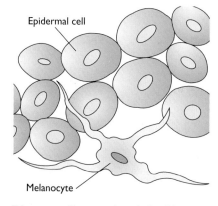

Epidermal cell

Melanocyte

Diagram to illustrate the relationship between pigment cells (melanocytes) and the epidermal cells. The melanocytes inject their melanin into the surrounding epidermal cells.

your genes. Curiously the number of pigment-producing cells (melanocytes) in the epidermis is the same whether you are a ginger-haired ruddy-complexioned Scot or a jet-black-skinned African from Ethiopia. The differences in the amount of melanin produced and the skin colour depend instead almost entirely on the *rate* of melanin pigment production.

Melanin is a substance composed of large complex molecules which are in effect polymers, and there are some slight and subtle variations in skin colour that are dependent on fairly small changes in the length and degree of folding of the melanin molecule. Skin colour is also influenced to a minor degree by whether it is produced in small or large clumps of pigment. And there is one other way in which the physical form of melanin may

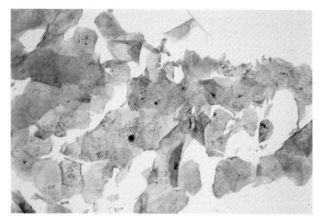

Many horn cells stained for the presence of melanin pigment.

alter skin colour. You may have noticed that your skin looks darker just an hour or two after being in the sun. This is not true tanning but the result of redistribution of melanin particles within the epidermal cells.

When melanin pigment is produced in the melanocytes, it doesn't just sit there but is injected by the spidery arms of the melanocytes into the neighbouring epidermal cells (see illustration on the bottom of page 26). Without this passing on of the pigment it cannot perform its protective function. The pigment is then carried upwards by the epidermal cells and is eventually lost at the surface in the horny cells of the stratum corneum. You may have noticed when you have been suntanned and your skin is slightly scaly that when the scale gets rubbed off it looks brownish. This is not just dirt but

the melanin in horny cells that has been carried up from the basal layer of the epidermis.

Some people's melanocytes seem very sluggish and unwilling to respond to the stimulus of the sun's ultraviolet rays. Usually such 'non-tanners' are fair-skinned and have red or auburn-coloured hair and blue or blue-green eyes. They burn very easily after exposure to the sun. Those with a Celtic ancestry—the Scots, Irish and Welsh—are particularly likely to have this type of complexion. Others with light complexions and blonde hair may sometimes burn but are also capable of tanning. As mentioned previously, there is a general rule that the darker your skin the more protected you are against damage from solar ultraviolet rays. However this doesn't always hold true; for example, I have quite a dark complexion but I burn quite easily. We just don't know all the factors that determine sun sensitivity.

It is quite useful to be able to classify people according to their sensitivity to the sun and the best simple scheme devised up to now is known as the Boston skin-type classification. It depends partially on the individual's answers to questions as to whether they burn or tan after sun exposure.

Type I   Always burns, never tans
Type II   Always burns, sometimes tans
Type III Sometimes burns, sometimes tans
Type IV   Never burns, always tans
Type V   Asiatic peoples from the Indian subcontinent and the Far East
Type VI   Black African and Caribbean peoples

Some unfortunate people are born with totally white skin and flaxen hair as a result of an inherited disorder of their melanocytes. Albinism is the name given to this disease, and the sufferers are known as albinos. If albinos don't protect themselves against the sun they can be most dreadfully burnt and damaged by solar UVR. In Nigeria there is a community of albinos who unfortunately tend to develop skin cancers in young adult life and sometimes die from these—all because they were born without a capacity for their skin to make melanin.

Apart from this inherited abnormality of melanocytes these pigment-producing cells are occasionally affected by disease acquired in adult life. One disorder in particular needs to be mentioned. Many readers will have heard of vitiligo, as it is quite a common problem. In this disease the melanocytes in one or several localized areas seem to 'go on strike'. We are not certain why this should be, but it does seem as though it is a particular kind of allergy to one's own melanocytes. The affected patches become white, and may be burnt after only a little exposure to the sun, although the surrounding normal skin is unaffected.

Increase in the degree of skin pigmentation (tanning) is sometimes seen without sun exposure. In fact when the skin becomes inflamed in a variety of skin disorders the affected area may darken during the healing phase. An increase in pigmentation is also sometimes observed at the site of persistent mechanical irritation or chemical injury. It seems that the melanocytes can be stimulated by many different sorts of injury, not just the injury from ultraviolet irradiation. Increased pigmentation due to abnormal production of melanin may also occur all over the body due to a hormone disorder or some other generalized metabolic problem.

Darkening of the skin is not always due to the production of more melanin. It is also due rarely to some other dark substance being dumped in the skin. Some drugs can cause the skin to pigment, although the pigmentation doesn't often look quite like suntan. For example, chlorpromazine, one of the drugs that has been used to treat psychiatric illnesses, can produce a curious dusky mauve-purple discolouration in the sun-exposed sites. An antibiotic called minocycline, and a drug used to treat irregular heart beats, amiodarone, are two other medications that can make the skin darken (see Chapter 4).

Site differences

We all know that the soles of our feet and our palms are covered by skin that looks, feels and behaves differently from skin elsewhere over the body. The thickness and toughness of the skin of the palms and soles give the protection necessary for these sites, and is in marked contrast to the thinness and delicacy of the facial skin. The stratum corneum of the sole is in the region of 0.5 mm thick, about 100 times thicker than the stratum corneum of the eyelid.

The thickness of the horny layer is just one way in which skin varies over different parts of the body. For example, the number and size of sweat glands and hair follicles differs markedly over the body surface. Similarly the number of small blood vessels, and their size, distribution and arrangement within the skin is characteristic for each part of the body. For example, the face has a large number of small blood vessels, some of which are quite near the surface. This is why the cheeks have that pink look to them and why the face flushes and blushes so easily.

Body sites at risk from the sun

Fashion, climate, social class and religion are just some of the things that influence which bits of the skin are continually exposed to the sun. Recently we have tried to study skin that had never (or only rarely) been sun exposed in young healthy adults. It was stunning to find that there were few staff or students that were suitable for our research. Most of the ones we asked had exposed most of their skin in the recent past on some sun-drenched beach or other.

All sorts of oddities in sun exposure crop up—such as the fact that drivers in Australia develop more sun damage on the arms by the driver's-side window, bald-headed men tend to develop the worst effects of sun exposure on the exposed scalp, women tend to develop small growths of the skin on the lower parts of the lower legs away from the shadows of their skirts, the tops of men's ears are sometimes badly affected by the sun but women's ears are not because they are protected by their hair. There are numerous other examples of differences in the sites of solar damage that depend on fashion and custom. The geography of the face means that some parts are badly damaged by the sun and other parts are not. The upper lip and the underside of the chin are rarely damaged because they are in the shade of the nose and chin respectively, while the forehead, bridge of the nose, the upper cheeks and the lower lip are prone to the more severe types of damage from the sun because they are exposed to the sun's rays without any natural protection.

Inflammation and repair

All kinds of injury may inflame the skin, from infection—by bacteria, viruses or fungi—to allergy. Sunburn is just such an injury. In any sort of inflammation the injury causing the problem is responsible for releasing chemical substances from the skin cells. These chemical substances make the blood vessels dilate so that there is a faster flow of blood in them. Fluid leaks out from these widened vessels so that the affected area becomes red from the increased supply of blood and swollen from the increased fluid. The swelling makes the area tender and painful. The chemical substances released also attract 'scavenger' white blood cells into the area to help get rid of any infection or unwanted foreign material. The white cells then also release chemicals which can damage the tissue and, when dead, can form pus in an abscess.

When damage occurs to the skin it repairs itself very efficiently and the process of healing is quite similar, regardless of whether the injury is caused by infection, a wound or severe sunburn. The cells of the skin move and divide to make good the loss, and if the injury is quite severe a scar forms. Healing is a very complex process as the tissues involved have to be 'informed' of what they have to do, and must be 'controlled' to prevent them doing what they are not supposed to do. Once again, chemical substances released from cells appear to control these processes.

4

Sunburn, sun sensitivity and sunstroke

Why should exposure to the sun have any harmful effect? The answer seems to be that the molecules that make up living cells are damaged and altered after being exposed to the UVR portion of the solar spectrum. The UVR raises the energy of the electrons around some atoms in these molecules so that they become 'excited'. In some molecules abnormal bonds form between the constituent atoms. Some proteins become denatured, i.e. so damaged they can no longer fulfil their usual function, and some molecules become oxidized, with a similar result.

At the centre of every mammalian cell there is a nucleus containing all the genetic information of that individual. The genetic information is stored on chromosomes, along which are placed the genes themselves. These genes consist of strands of a complex substance called deoxyribonucleic acid, or DNA for short. One of the targets for damage caused by UVR is the DNA itself. If severe enough, the damage sustained by the nuclear DNA will cause the cell to die. Lesser degrees of damage can in fact be even more threatening to the individual, for if there is permanent alteration to the nuclear DNA it could lead to some types of skin cancer.

Particular parts of the solar spectrum may have special biological effects. This is because some molecules appear to be able to absorb the energy of solar radiation at these particular wavelengths. As pointed out in Chapter 2, it is the UVR portion of the solar spectrum that seems to have the most impact on biological systems, although not all the wavelengths in the UVR range are important in this way—the shortwave UVR known as UVC never reaches the earth's surface as it is filtered out by the ozone layer and the atmosphere. It seems that the most damage to the skin is due to the UVR band that ranges from 280 to 320 nanometres. This is the band known as UVB, or the 'sunburn band'.

Sunburn

Anyone who has had a good dose of sunburn tries to avoid being burnt again. I am ashamed to say that I can confirm just how unpleasant bad sunburn can be—but then I was young and ignorant and no-one pointed out how silly it was to sunbathe at the height of the midday sun, even in the UK.

After receiving the UVR dose that causes the burn, a series of changes

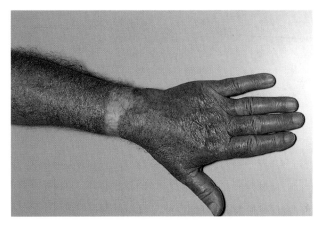

Sunburn. Notice the area shielded by a watch has not been burnt.

take place in the skin. For the first few hours very little happens. Then about four or six hours afterwards (usually it is just as you are getting ready for your evening meal!) the areas of skin that have been burnt feel hot, prickly and tense, and the skin looks slightly pink. As the evening wears on you feel increasingly uncomfortable and, depending on how bad the problem is, sleep may be quite difficult. The following morning the affected areas are bright red and acutely uncomfortable and the sore skin won't tolerate anything rubbing over it or sudden changes in temperature. Having a bath can be a major problem, with the victim only very slowly allowing the water to touch the sore parts of the skin. The sharpness of the line between the burnt and the unburnt areas of skin depends on the clothing worn. If, as is

often the case, an opaque thickish swimming costume is worn, there is a sharp line between the reddened sore area and the white unburnt areas beneath the costume. If, on the other hand, a flimsy cotton garment has been the only protection for the unburnt skin then the distinction between the affected and unaffected areas may be much less dramatic because the rays penetrate the thin cotton to some extent and may cause some pinkness on the covered sites.

Obviously the severity of the problem will depend on the amount of radiation received and the inherent protection and sensitivity of the skin itself. The skin's own system of protection is examined in Chapter 3. It will also depend on the area of skin that has been exposed. In the worst cases, where the back and front of the trunk as well as the limbs and face are involved, the afflicted individual may be quite unwell and, apart from the extreme discomfort in the skin, may feel dreadful and have a fever. They may also be dehydrated because water is lost through the skin, which may become blistered and moist.

After a few days the redness and soreness die away and the peeling begins. It is as though you have been sprayed with a plastic film. It bubbles in places and just peels off in others. The top part of the skin can simply be pulled off, and we all seem to take a ghoulish delight in peeling off as large a piece as possible. The peeling phase lasts up to five days and leaves the skin beneath either slightly pink or slightly tanned.

What is the explanation for all these changes? We don't know all the answers but in the past few years the situation has been made much clearer. The UVR mostly affects the epidermis and in fact very little of the radiation actually penetrates down into the upper dermis. Although the whole epidermis is damaged, there is an odd spotty kind of distribution of dead epidermal cells in the middle of the epidermis. These are known appropriately enough as sunburn cells. The damaged epidermal cells release chemical substances that set in motion the series of events that make the skin inflamed. Some of these chemical 'mediator' substances are known as prostaglandins and seem to be responsible for the widening of the small blood vessels of the skin and the redness that this causes. The increased blood supply to the burnt

area also allows more tissue fluid and white cells to accumulate in the area so that the area becomes swollen. During recovery from the sudden injury caused by the blast of solar radiation the epidermis suddenly thickens up, due to the cells dividing more rapidly.

Light sensitivity

What has been described above is ordinary sunburn, when the sun's UVR reaches the skin in sufficient amounts to override the melanin defence system. In some circumstances the same kind of sunburn reaction can occur after only a tiny amount of UVR has been received, and this is known as light sensitivity. Light sensitivity may be due to the skin being made more vulnerable to UVR by a drug, either taken by mouth or put on the skin in a cream, lotion or ointment, or it may be due to a disease of some kind.

Drug-induced light sensitivity

The list of drugs that can cause light sensitivity (or photosensitivity as it is sometimes called) is horrifyingly long, but usually this effect is an infrequent accompaniment of taking one of the drugs. The very useful group of

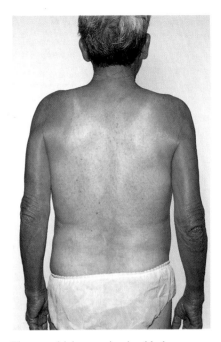

Photosensitivity reaction in elderly man who took tetracycline. Notice that where his vest covered his back the skin is not red.

actual nail begins to separate from the nail bed on which it usually rests. This is known technically by the tongue-twister term of onycholysis—when it is caused by drug-induced light sensitivity it is known as photo-onycholysis.

In some cases the drug-induced light sensitivity has particular characteristics due to the special effects of the drug in combination with UVR. For example, some drugs used to treat mental disorders have been found to cause a curious purplish discolouration in light-exposed areas of skin. The drug mostly to blame for this problem is known as Largactil. It is much less used now than it used to be so that there are fewer 'purple people' attending psychiatric clinics than previously! The reason for the odd discolouration appears to be that under the influence of UVR a chemical derivative of Largactil joins on to the melanin (see page 26) in skin tissues.

Another type of drug-induced light sensitivity causes blistering of the skin. Nalidixic acid is one of the drugs known to cause this problem; this is used to treat infections of the kidney and bladder.

Drugs and other chemicals applied directly to the skin can also be the cause of a photosensitivity reaction. One of the most frequent offenders in this way is the group of substances known as the psoralens. These occur in a variety of plants and fruits whose photosensitizing properties have been recognized for many hundreds of years. The type of photosensitization produced characteristically causes

tetracycline antibiotic drugs can cause photosensitivity as can some drugs used in heart diseases (such as amiodarone) and drugs used to treat some mental disorders (see below). The tetracyclines are used for all sorts of common diseases including bronchitis, sinusitis and severe acne. One curious point about the light sensitivity caused by the tetracyclines is that it is sometimes accompanied by an odd deformity of the fingernails. In this the brown pigmentation after the redness subsides. This tanning effect has been employed by some manufacturers of skin-care products, saying that their products cause tanning without burning. Even if tanning was a desirable objective and the products did in fact promote tanning without visible burning, it seems highly unlikely to me that tanning could occur without any type of epidermal damage.

The photosensitization caused by the psoralens is the basis of a form of treatment (see page 77) for the chronic scaling skin condition called psoriasis. This special treatment relies on the combined effect of psoralens and long-wavelength UVR (UVA). The psoralens are given either by mouth as tablets or in a liquid application as a lotion or bath (see Chapter 8).

Light sensitivity due to psoralens also occurs after contact with some fruits and plants or extracts of these. I suppose the classic example is that seen on the backs of young men and women who romp in meadows containing lots of giant hogweed. The juice of the crushed plant plus the sun causes a light sensitivity rash in some rather embarrassing places. It is also seen in blameless middle-aged men who contact with the crushed giant hogweed merely stems from mowing the lawn! This type of rash is called phytophotodermatitis by dermatologists (phyto meaning to do with a plant, and photo meaning to do with light).

So far I have only mentioned sunburn, blistering and various pigmentations being caused by the combination of chemical substances and UVR from the sun. Another quite common way in which the skin may react to the toxic effects of the 'sun and substance' combination is by a type of eczema (another name for dermatitis). In the late 1950s and early 1960s a particular sort of dermatitis was noticed in some patients. It was confined to the light-exposed parts of the skin and the sudden appearance of the disorder made the whole thing very mysterious. Some fairly impressive clinical detective work soon revealed that the cause was a group of antimicrobial chemical substances added to soaps and toiletries to make them (and people) smell better. The group of chemicals which have this light-sensitizing effect is known as the halogenated salicylanilides, and the particular culprit was one of these, called tetrachlorosalicylanilide, which was added to a particular soap.

There are many similar examples of rashes of one sort and another being caused by the photosensitizing effect of a drug used in treatment or a chemical in the environment, and obviously I can't describe them all, but I hope that I have included enough to make the reader aware of this kind of sun-induced problem.

Other rashes caused by the sun

Some skin disorders are caused by or aggravated by exposure to the sun without being provoked by drugs or by substances that come in contact with the skin. We know more about some of these than others. In one group of diseases there are abnormalities in the way that the body makes certain parts of the haemoglobin molecule found in the red blood cells. These disorders are known as the porphyrias, and in the different sorts of porphyria normal substances are produced in greatly abnormal amounts in the body and these then act in the same way as the photosensitizing drugs discussed above. These substances are known as the porphyrins. The porphyrias are mostly, but not exclusively, disorders that are inherited, and because they are such an interesting group of light-provoked diseases I will spend a little time describing some of the different types.

Probably the most notorious type of porphyria is the type that may have affected King George III, although on the whole the evidence for this seems somewhat shaky. Another tragic, though interesting, form of porphyria is the inherited disorder known as erythropoietic porphyria. This is the disease that is supposed to have given birth to the legend of the werewolf. This particular abnormality of porphyrin metabolism leads to the most remarkable photosensitivity, starting in infancy, which eventually causes dreadful scarring and deformity. There is also a tendency for abnormal growth of hair in the affected areas. The facial scars and deformity and the excess hairiness

can give a bizarre appearance to these unfortunate individuals. This, combined with their fear of going out during the day because of the risk of further light-induced damage, seems to have generated the idea that those afflicted with this disease gave rise to the legend of the werewolf. To add to the oddity of their appearance, their teeth take up the abnormal porphyrin and fluoresce a rather striking red colour when UVR is shone on them. This frightening disorder is luckily extremely rare.

A somewhat less rare variety of porphyria is known as porphyria cutanea tarda. There seems to be some type of inherited tendency to this disorder, even though it doesn't come on until into middle age, but it is not clear cut. What seems to be more certain is that most of the patients affected by this malady have a liver problem and often drink to excess. The disorder usually declares itself with blistering on the light exposed areas, particularly on the backs of the hands and the forehead. The affected areas of skin become scarred and pigmented and may also become excessively hairy. In one group of patients from Turkey with this disease, the problem started after they ate food contaminated with the poison hexachlorobenzene (normally used for its antimicrobial qualities).

There is yet another type of light sensitivity seen with an uncommon type of porphyria known as erythropoietic protoporphyria. In this inherited disease the particular porphyrin abnormality results in painful red swellings in the skin of the light-exposed areas. These develop a few minutes after being out in the sun and last for some hours afterwards. They look like the condition known popularly as hives and by doctors as urticaria. To make things more complicated, some patients have an urticaria type of rash if they go out in the sun which is not due to porphyria!

Porphyria represents a group of disorders where we know quite a lot about the nature of the underlying problem, but regrettably this is not the case for several other light-provoked disorders. I won't describe each one in great detail but I think that it is reasonable to include a few general comments. Most of these disorders are recurrent; that is, they start each year some time in March or April when the intensity of solar UVR increases. Also they tend to last for several years. The rashes in these disorders are predominantly on the light-exposed areas of skin but may not be completely confined to them, so that they can be very difficult for even an experienced dermatologist to diagnose. Mostly the affected individuals are moderately sensitive to the sun but some unlucky patients are so sensitive that they are virtually condemned to live in dimly-lit rooms and are only able to go out at night. The reason for this is that, while usually it is a fairly limited part of the solar spectrum that causes these light-induced rashes, with longwave UVR being particularly blameworthy, in the very sensitive patients it seems that they may also be sensitive to visible light.

Apart from skin diseases that are actually caused by exposure to the sun there are also several skin disorders that are aggravated or precipitated by exposure to the sun. One of these disorders is known as lupus erythematosus. This condition is either confined as a rash to the skin or can cause an unpleasant generalized illness in which there is fever and arthritis, amongst other things. Either of these forms of the disorder can be aggravated by exposure to solar UVR and patients with the disease should be quite careful to avoid the sun.

Even ordinary infantile eczema may be aggravated by being out in the sun, although this only applies to a small number of patients and many actually seem to improve in the sun. The same is true for psoriasis. Most patients with psoriasis improve in the sun; in fact some form or other of UVR is a frequently-used form of treatment for this disease (see Chapter 8). There are a few, though, that actually worsen after being exposed to the sun. I can remember at least two patients who first developed psoriasis when and where they became sunburnt.

Sweat rash

Different people mean different things by sweat rash, and I don't want anyone to run away with the idea that the term means one specific thing. The most frequent type of sweat rash develops in hot weather in the groins of those with 'generous' thighs. A story I am frequently told is that the rash develops during a summer holiday at the seaside. The explanation is that becoming hot and sweaty on the beach in the usual swimsuit leads to chafing of the skin of one thigh against the other. The redness and soreness persist unless efforts are made to stay cool for a bit and normal clothes are worn so that there is less friction on the skin. The same kind of problem can develop in the armpits, but this is seen less often. A similar condition can develop in elderly overweight women in hot humid weather, regardless of the clothes they are wearing. The rash in this group is found not only in the groins and armpits but in all the other folds and creases of the skin as well. A particularly awkward spot that often develops a sweat rash of this type is the skin under the breasts. In the worst cases the sweat rash becomes infected and the reddened area develops pus spots and becomes oozy. Often the infection is due to a yeast-type of fungus called *Candida*, and the condition is known as thrush.

Another type of sweat rash is due to the horny surface layer around the openings of the sweat ducts becoming swollen, resulting in the blockage of the sweat gland. If the sweat gland keeps on working even though its pore is blocked the end of the duct becomes distended out into a little clear fluid-filled blob. As these little blobs are as clear as a crystal, the name of miliaria crystallina has been used to describe the condition. This is really quite common in the summer, especially in feverish infants. Itchiness and slight soreness are the main complaints but the condition usually rapidly subsides if the affected person keeps cool. Uncommonly, the blockage to the sweat glands is deeper within the skin or the affected glands become infected. The rash then looks lumpy and red and is more painful and uncomfortable.

It used to be said that a particular sort of eczema on the hands was due to a disorder of sweat glands and was a sort of sweat rash. This disorder is marked by the appearance of multitudes of tiny clear fluid-filled blisters on the palms and sides of the fingers. These were thought to be due to blocked sweat ducts and this opinion seemed reinforced by the fact that the disorder often worsens in the hot weather. In fact the condition, which goes by the odd name of cheiropompholyx, really has little to do with sweating and is just an odd type of eczema.

Sunstroke and heat exhaustion

With the tame summers that we often have in the UK one wouldn't imagine that there is much of a chance of developing problems such as heat exhaustion or sunstroke. Somehow, though, a few people always seem to manage it.

The two conditions are really quite different. Sunstroke or heat stroke is quite a dangerous condition in which the body's usual protection against overheating fails. Obviously it mainly occurs in very hot weather and may be precipitated by a fever. It is most common in athletes who overdo it or in soldiers who have been poorly trained. The body temperature rises to biologically unacceptable levels and 'all systems fail'. Heat exhaustion is quite different and, although very unpleasant, is not quite so dangerous. With this condition the main problem is one of loss of body fluid and salt from sweating. This causes difficulties with the circulation and blood pressure and can lead to collapse.

A very interesting adaptation takes place in the skin in hot, humid climates. When someone travels from a cool climate to somewhere tropical they have a high rate of sweating for the first two or three weeks. With acclimatization the rate of sweating decreases and there is less danger of a fluid and salt problem.

Testing for light sensitivity

This section outlines some of the tests performed to reach or confirm a diagnosis of a skin disorder caused by exposure to light. In fact for the most part 'light' sensitivity is an improper term to use, and UVR sensitivity would be more appropriate, as very few disorders show sensitivity to visible light. Most of the tests are peformed with artificially-produced UVR from special lamps.

Basically there are three main types of lamp. There is the ordinary sunlamp type, which may be satisfactory for some purposes. The problem with this sort of apparatus is that it doesn't give out radiation in the UVR spectrum which is continuous like the sun, but only emits UVR at certain wavelengths or wavebands, dependent on the lamps. As one of the wavebands emitted is in the sunburn wavelength range, i.e. 290–310 nm, they can be used to determine the degree of sun sensitivity present. The minimal length of exposure required to produce pinkness of the skin some 12–16 hours after irradiation, that persists for a few days, is determined. Not unexpectedly, this is known as the minimal erythema dose (MED), which will of course depend on the strength of the lamp and on the distance the skin is away from the lamp. It is usual to shine the UVR onto several small patches of skin for different times, shielding all areas but the one to be irradiated each time, so that the first one which causes the persistent redness can be identified easily.

Sometimes a small patch of skin will be irradiated to see if it provokes the disorder being described. If a rash appears at the test site it may be sampled to confirm the diagnosis microscopically. Another sort of test uses the second type of lamp—the solar simulator (see Chapter 2). Essentially this is an expensive bit of apparatus which copies the solar UVR spectrum. This is particularly useful in what is called photo patch testing, where the suspected substance (see pages 33–35) is placed on the skin and the area is then irradiated to see if it brings out the rash.

The third sort of testing lamp used is quite complicated. It is called a monochromator, and is able to irradiate small areas of skin with UVR at any particular wavelength required. Many disorders in which 'light' plays a role are sensitive to a narrow waveband of UVR only, and the monochromator can be used to determine if there is sensitivity and, if so, to which particular wavelength. For example, in the porphyrias there is a special sensitivity to UVR at the odd wavelength of 404 nm.

5

Ageing and the sun

The subject of ageing has become extremely important in Western society. Increased affluence and improved social conditions, as well as the development of antibiotics and other life-saving drugs, have resulted in increasing longevity. We are now witnessing a population explosion—in those over 80! The idea of getting old is extremely distasteful for most of us, and the development of age-retarding, age-reversing and age-disguising cosmetics has become a growth industry. Biological research into the process of ageing and how to defeat its effects has also burgeoned in recent years. It is quite evident that no-one wants to look old.

What is ageing?

First of all we ought to be clear by what we mean by 'looking old'. For most of us the process of growing old means such things as going grey, losing one's teeth, becoming shorter and bent, and developing wrinkles and other changes in the skin. The alterations in the skin are of major importance to the perception of ageing and, as sun exposure plays such a central role in the process, we need to examine these alterations in some detail.

It is important that we distinguish three types of ageing - chronological ageing, intrinsic ageing and extrinsic ageing. Chronological ageing is merely the 'ticking of the clock', the passing of the years, which no-one can prevent. Intrinsic ageing describes the inevitable changes built into tissues that occur with the passage of time and which are not influenced by disease or external stimuli of any kind. However, when the body's tissues and organs are repeatedly or persistently injured by some external agency they gradually break down, and this is the process I refer to as extrinsic ageing. Intrinsic and extrinsic ageing together cause the individual to have an 'apparent age'.

Although these three types of ageing may occur together, they often seem to occur at different rates. We all know spry elderly individuals of over 70 who look and behave much younger than their years. And of course there are those unfortunates who look tired and aged at 35. Part of the reason for this appears to be that the intrinsic ageing process, whatever it is, varies enormously between different people. This makes research into ageing extremely tricky!

Sailors, farmers, roofers and others who have to work outdoors all the time tend to have a battered look in later life. Their apparent age is greater than their chronological age and is due to the extrinsic ageing effect of the damage sustained from the elements. Of course we all differ as to how much we are exposed to assault from the vagaries of the climate, and to some extent this will determine how old we look. Unfortunately the problem is more complicated than that. The amount of damage to the skin tissues from the environment also depends on the efficiency of the skin's protective and repair mechanisms (see Chapter 3). This means that a dusky brown farmer from North Africa will not appear aged compared to a red or fair-haired individual from northern Europe, given the same degree of climatic exposure.

Skin ageing

Having learnt that ageing is a very complex issue, let me try to describe the clinical changes that take place in the skin with the passing of the years, and then be more specific about whether each change is the result of intrinsic or extrinsic ageing.

As the years roll by your skin becomes thinner in all body sites. For example, the thickness of the dermis of the forearm in a normal man aged 18 to 40 is about 1.1 mm. In a man of 80 this thins to about 0.75 mm. Women's skin starts off somewhat thinner—the skin on the forearm of a woman 18 to 40 years old would be about 0.9 mm

thick. Thinning of the skin due to age is proportionately less, and, for example, at the age of 80 forearm-skin thickness in a woman is only a little less than in a man of the same age.

Apart from the thickness or thinness of the skin, its mechanical properties alter markedly with age. Skin becomes less elastic and resilient in the elderly. Pinch up a fold of skin on the back of the hand. It's actually quite hard to pick up much of a fold at all in a young, fit person. The older the person pinched, the longer it takes for the fold to settle back again. In fact it is quite different in severely sun-damaged individuals compared to a non-sun-damaged person—but we will come back to this point later. The 'stiffness' of skin actually increases with age, although it may appear otherwise. The droopiness that can be seen over the abdomen or around the upper arms of overweight elderly people is more a function of the laxity and increased amount of fat in the tissues immediately under the skin than due to laxness in the skin itself.

The reason for this change in the stretchability and toughness of skin with age is quite complex from the chemical point of view. It is due to the alterations in the collagen of the dermis (see Chapter 3), in which this fibrous protein becomes less soluble because more chemical links are formed between the molecules. In addition, the jelly-like material (ground substance) between the dermal collagen fibres almost disappears during the ageing process.

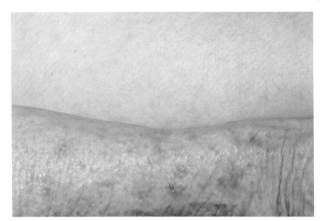

The photodamaged forearm of this elderly lady is very different from her normally protected abdominal skin. Note that the exposed skin shows mottled pigmentation and seems thicker and rougher than the smooth, pale skin of the abdomen.

Furthermore, the surface of the skin changes strikingly in old age. The changes are much more marked in skin of sun-exposed sites, but are also present on protected skin. Generally speaking, old skin feels and looks drier than younger skin. It seems slightly rougher and has lost that bloom of youth. Actually there is not too much evidence that there is less moisture in the skin, although there is no doubt that the skin certainly looks as though it is drier. The dry appearance is often accompanied by some itchiness, and also by chapping of the skin. These problems are much worse in cold weather and much, much worse in climates that have a low relative humidity. The north-east of the United States is notorious for this sort of problem and it is made especially bad by the drying effect of the central heating systems used there.

The reason for this drying and scaling of elderly skin is quite mysterious. We know that the epidermis thins with increasing age and at the same time the keratinocytes shrink in size and the corneocytes (which produce the horny outer layer of skin) become longer and wider. Presumably changes in the function of the epidermis and stratum corneum also take place which could account for the effects at the skin surface.

Wrinkling

Interestingly, the surface markings on the skin surface become less prominent

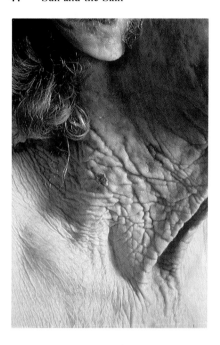

Gross solar elastotic degeneration affecting the neck in a late middle-aged lady of Celtic derivation. She claimed not to have had much sun exposure.

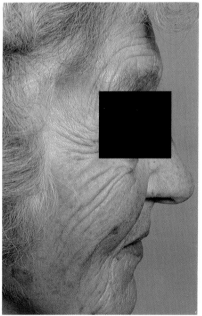

Fine lines and wrinkles all over the skin of the face due to solar elastotic degenerative change.

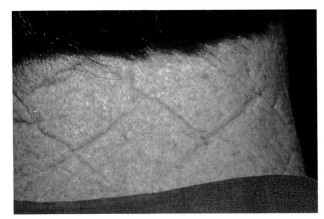

Typical changes on the neckline of an ex-sailor. Redness and the lining gives rise to the term 'red neck' and is also seen in agricultural workers, roofers and all those who spend much time out of doors.

in old age. This effect is very much more marked in sun-exposed sites—and is quite independent of wrinkling. Wrinkling itself is mainly seen on sun-exposed sites—particularly the face and neck—and is believed to be due chiefly to the effects of the sun on the dermal connective tissue; the more you are sun-exposed the more wrinkles you develop. So, going back to what has been said at the beginning of this chapter with regard to ageing, wrinkling is an extrinsic ageing effect. Of course if you are dark-skinned you are much less likely to be sun-damaged and much less likely to be wrinkled. Look around at the older members of the white-skinned communities in Australia, South Africa or the southern states of the USA, and it becomes obvious that wrinkling is strongly associated with sun exposure.

Wrinkling seems to be the result of changes in the texture and mechanical properties of connective tissue after it has been severely damaged by solar UVR. The alteration that the sun produces in the dermal connective tissue has been copied by shining artificial UV radiation on to the skin of animals and, all things considered, we now feel that there is good evidence that the sun is responsible for the changes we observe. The changes in the dermis due to solar damage are known by the term solar elastotic degeneration or, more simply, as solar elastosis. This odd name was given because the damaged tissue takes on many of the properties of normal elastic tissue (which, you will remember from page 24, does *not* give the skin its elastic properties). Some research workers have gone so far as to say that the

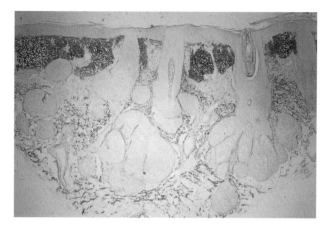

Photomicrograph of skin section showing dark mauve areas beneath the epidermis demonstrating the elastotic degeneration to the dermal connective tissue.

abnormal dermal connective tissue is actually newly-formed elastic tissue replacing the older collagen. From a practical point of view, it really doesn't matter whether this is true or not because, regardless of the exact nature of the abnormal tissue, it causes the affected skin to lose its normal strength and stretchability.

A specimen of skin from an area of sun damage can easily be distinguished down the microscope by the presence of this solar elastosis. The sun-damaged dermis can be made out as a band just below the epidermis. The thickness and density of the band depends on the severity of the damage. Even in the comparatively sunless UK it is usual to find some traces of solar elastosis in facial skin in adults over the age of 25. The damaged dermal tissue can be made to stand out by staining the speci-

men with special stains that show up elastic tissue under the microscope.

Brown spots and warts

Wrinkling is just one of the signs of apparent ageing due to solar elastosis. Aged skin may also show other more subtle changes in skin colour. On covered parts the skin becomes slightly paler due to a drop in the numbers of pigment cells (melanocytes, see Chapter 3) and a lessening of their pigment-producing activity. This decreased pigmentation is not really noticeable on sun-exposed skin, and instead on markedly sun-damaged skin there may be a faint pasty lemon or sallow tinge due to the solar elastosis itself.

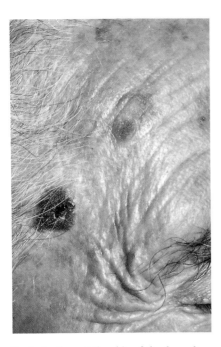

Senile lentigos at the side of the face of an elderly man.

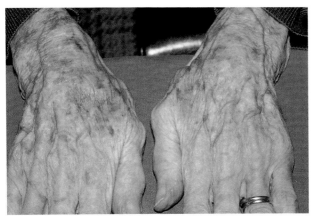

Senile lentigos on the backs of the hands of a late-middle-aged woman.

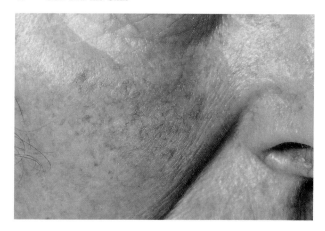

'Broken veins' on the cheek of a man with photodamaged skin.

Flat or slightly raised brown patches occur over the backs of the hands and over the face in the elderly. These benign discolourations are unsightly and unpopular with their owners. They are known medically as senile lentigos, popularly as liver spots, and more colourfully by the French as *les medallions de cimetière* (cemetery medals). These brown marks are due almost entirely to persistent sun exposure and damage to the pigment cells in the exposed skin. Recent studies show that although they all look similar the brown spots may actually represent one of several minor abnormalities. Many similar spots sometimes appear over the back and chest and, where they do, they often become quite raised up and develop a hard, irregular warty surface. These are quite harmless seborrhoeic warts, but have to be distinguished from other, less benign, spots (see Chapter 6).

Broken veins

Because dermal connective tissue affected by solar elastosis isn't as tough or as resilient as normal connective tissue, the blood vessels that cross it don't have their usual mechanical support. This allows these blood vessels to widen and become visible at the skin surface. These visible blood vessels are known technically as telangiectasia, and are popularly known as 'broken veins'. If you look at the backs of the forearms and on the backs of the hands of elderly folk who are quite sun-battered you often see crimson patches which look like fresh bruises. These localized patches are called senile purpura, and are also the result of solar elastosis. We think of these patches as being caused by the widened unsupported blood vessels in the abnormal dermis being easily damaged by any slight knock or bump and then bleeding slightly into the skin. Because the ability of all the cells and tissues to repair themselves is somewhat slowed down in the elderly, these senile-purpura type of bruises take a long time to fade away.

Sometimes the extent of the solar damage is so great that the skin is actually slightly thickened by the abnormal solar elastotic degenerative change and seems slightly lumpy. On the neck, when combined with wrinkling and the faint pasty lemon-yellow tinge mentioned above, this gives an appearance not very different from chicken skin! Odd types of scars also appear on the backs of severely sun-damaged forearms. These scars are sometimes star-shaped or shaped like boomerangs. No-one knows exactly why they come but they don't seem to be due to any significant mechanical injury and are strongly associated with the presence of solar elastosis.

Inflammation and immunity

All types of inflammation seem to be less intense in elderly skin. Sunburn reactions are less dramatic and skin reactions to irritating chemicals are also less marked. There are probably many different reasons why inflammatory responses are dulled in old age. Diminished ability of the blood vessels to widen and decreased mobility of some of the blood's white cells account for some of the decreased vigour of inflammation. There is also a slackening of the body's immune defences in general, so that our responses to infection are weaker in old age.

The Langerhans cells in the skin (see page 19) are a recently-discovered important component of our immune defence system. It seems that these cells pick up potentially dangerous substances that penetrate the skin. Having picked them up, they 'process' them and pass them on so that an immunological attack can be mounted against them—that is how, say, nickel allergy or poison ivy dermatitis arises. In old age the numbers of Langerhans cells in the epidermis drops. In fact it is true to say that elderly people become less easily 'allergic' to things that they contact than when they were young. More interesting is the fact that the number and function of Langerhans cells dramatically drops after exposure of the skin to solar UVR. Indeed it has been demonstrated in experiments that it is more difficult to develop an allergy after UVR exposure. It has even been proposed that artificial UVR may be a reasonable treatment for this type of allergy.

The decrease in Langerhans cells may be important in one other major respect and that is in the development of skin cancer. It is thought by some researchers that our immune defences help protect us against cancer and when these defences are depressed for any reason, growths have a greater chance of developing. Obviously we are now getting into a complicated scientific area; in any case, we can safely put off discussing it now as it is the subject of the next chapter.

Treatment

It must be admitted right from the start that, up to now, drug treatments for the effects of persistent sun exposure on the skin have been either ineffectual or unproven. I don't want to appear too pessimistic, but it seems unlikely that we will see any major break-through within the next 10 years or so as far as ageing itself is concerned. However, there is one group of drugs that looks quite promising to some scientists for counteracting some of the effects of chronic sun damage. These drugs are known as the reti-noids and are rather like vitamin A.

One of this group of drugs, known as vitamin A acid or tretinoin (all-*trans*-retinoic acid, to give its full name) has been used successfully in creams and lotions in the treatment of acne since 1970. In the past few years, however, research has been published suggesting that the same drug can also stimulate repair of skin damage caused by the sun. In one very interesting series of experiments, damage caused by UVR from sunlamps to the dermal connec-tive tissue of mice was repaired after treatment with the vitamin A acid pre-paration, whereas in untreated mice the repair did not occur. Studies in patients and volunteers confirm these laboratory findings. Although the improvement takes several months of continuous use and the repair falls short of com-pletely restoring youthful skin, there is no doubt that quite substantial clinical improvement occurs. There is a reduc-tion in the fine lines on the skin, the patchy pigmentation decreases and the skin colour improves with the restora-tion of a healthier pink hue. The max-imum degree of improvement seems to occur after about 9 months of use and to maintain this degree of improvement it is necessary to continue treatment although this may be less frequently— say twice per week. Most work has been done with creams containing vita-min A acid but similar results have also been obtained with other drugs of the same class (retinoids). (I will mention the retinoids again in the next chapter when we tackle the question of treat-ments for skin cancer.)

Having started off this section by describing one group of drugs that might work we must also mention some other approaches to the pro-blem. Careful use of efficient sunsc-reens every time one goes out into the sun has been suggested. This should prevent any further damage and (it is said) should allow the natural repair processes to replace the damaged tis-sue. Even if the theory is right and it was possible, by the obsessive use of really efficient sun-barrier creams, to prevent any further damage, it would still take a very long time before any improvement occurred. All repair pro-cesses are slowed in the elderly and although sunscreens should be used to slow down or prevent further damage, it doesn't seem likely that they will catch on as a form of treatment.

Various 'repair creams' have been promoted to repair the damage to the skin caused by UV radiation. Some of these contain repair enzymes obtained from bacteria which, if they were able to work in human tissues and were able to penetrate the skin, theoretically could help replace altered genetic material in sun-damaged skin cells. Unfortunately there is no good evidence that they actually do improve the sun-damaged skin after use—and they are very expensive! The brown marks on the backs of the hands and sometimes over the face are unsightly and not very easy to disguise. Creams and lotions have been produced to bleach these; mostly they contain a substance known as hydroquinone which has the effect of interfering with melanin production.

What else are we left with? There remain all the wrinkle-removing and blemish-reducing anti-ageing cosmetic products. I cannot comment on each and every one, even if the space allowed, but some general comments are needed. Many of the cosmetic companies have evolved a high technology to detect particularly beneficial properties in their products. Most of the perceived benefit from the use of this class of cosmetics is to do with their emollient, soothing, smoothing and softening effects on the skin surface.

These products certainly do these things to varying degrees of efficiency, as well as with a considerable amount of charm and promised romance. What they cannot do, despite the obvious implications in their advertisements, is put collagen or elastin or any other tissue component back into a damaged skin. 'New collagen' or 'elastin' may have super cosmetic qualities in that they make the creams and lotions look and feel good, but it seems unlikely that they have any other effect as there is no good evidence that the large molecules of these compounds are actually absorbed into the skin. Wrinkles do seem to be less prominent after the use of some anti-wrinkle preparations, but I suspect that the apparent benefit is short-lived and simply due to the smoothing emollient action of the preparations.

Finally, it is worth warning against organ and plant extracts. They are often promoted with tremendous skill, but the evidence for their effectiveness is usually not forthcoming. It may sound paradoxical, but some of the 'natural' products and extracts used are often less safe than completely artificial chemical substances. Think of the sting in nettles and the dermatitis that can result from contact with some plants and you will realize that living things may contain quite harmful substances. 'Artificial' substances are often chosen because testing has demonstrated that they are quite safe to use.

Surgical and destructive treatments

The term 'face-lift' is so well-known that it has taken on a general meaning to describe any renovative procedure. There is no doubt that the various tricks employed in such plastic surgery are quite effective; double chins are reduced to their original singularity, eye bags are emptied and flattened, and wrinkle lines erased. It is certainly helpful for droopiness of facial and neck skin, but it can do little for the close-up appearance of the skin itself.

Chemical peeling with various destructive reagents such as phenol and trichloroacetic acid has been used for some time to try to rid the skin of superficial blemishes and fine lines. The success obtained is variable and quite unpredictable, and it is certainly a technique only for those with training and experience. More recently 'peeling' techniques using glycolic acid have become quite popular and may be helpful in the hands of experts, who claim that their treatments improve the appearance of sun-damaged skin.

6

Skin cancer

Luckily we have moved out of the era when cancer was a taboo subject and when any attempt at intelligent discussion of the disease only succeeded in generating fear. Now we recognize that cancer is not a single disease but a collection of quite different disorders that range from leukaemia to brain tumours. The only common feature of all the different forms of cancer is that the underlying problem is a disorderly, unregulated and irregular growth of some of the body's many tissues. Many of the provoking causes for the different types of cancer are unknown, but quite a few are known and seem specific to each of the particular forms of the disease. For example, we know that smoking is a potent cause of lung cancer and of no other form of the disease, although it may play some role in bladder and stomach cancer. Radiation from X-rays and from sources of radioactivity seem preferentially to cause leukaemia. Similarly, we know that the tendency to develop some forms of bowel cancer is inherited. Although there may be basic faults in the regulation of cell activities that go wrong in cancer of all types, the provoking agencies for the various forms of the disease are different.

Cancer, or neoplastic disease as it is sometimes known, causes problems in the body and may ultimately kill because the new disordered tissue produced disturbs the normal tissues in some way or interferes with a body function. For example, lung cancer causes blockage of the bronchial passages and interferes with the essential process of breathing. Apart from the abnormal 'growth' interfering, because of its bulk or because it damages normal tissues by infiltrating them, cancerous tissue may spread through the body by cancer cells invading small blood vessels and 'hitching a ride' to other sites in the body. This process is known as metastasis and is the really dangerous part of cancer.

We sometimes talk about 'benign' and 'malignant' tumours when we discuss cancer. The kinds of processes I have described above, such as metastasis and infiltration of normal tissue, would be called malignant. When neither metastasis nor tissue infiltration occurs, but there is merely a slow growth of the abnormal tissue, a benign tumour results which usually does not cause much in the way of medical problems. There are many sorts of benign tumour in the skin; in fact they are so common and so harmless for the most part that they are not thought of as being tumours at all. Ordinary warts that children develop on their hands, feet or faces are small tumours stimulated by a particular sort of virus. The pigmented moles that we all have on our skin are also a sort of benign tumour.

Apart from benign and malignant tumours, we need to recognize one other type of growth; that is, a growth that is not yet malignant but if left could become malignant. Not illogically, we call such growths pre-malignant. These have a particular importance as far we we are concerned because they can usually be quite easily detected on the skin and then treated.

It used to be thought that the diagnosis of cancer was a death sentence. It should be emphasized that this is no longer the case. The outlook for patients with cancer is really very much improved, and many patients are completely cured of their disease. Of course it depends very much on the particular type of neoplastic disease present, but it is still true to say that with new drugs, new surgical techniques and the improved understanding of the disease, the survival rates for all types of cancer have dramatically improved since the mid-1960s.

Skin cancer

If you refer back to Chapter 3 you will see that the skin is quite a complex structure and consists of a large number of different tissues that are bound together to function as one complex organ. Neoplastic disease can affect any of the different cell types of the skin, and the particular cell type from

which the growth arises will determine the way the neoplasm or tumour behaves and its clinical appearance.

The surface of the skin is made up of a supple horny layer produced by the epidermis beneath. Tumours of this epidermis are really very common. The most common, I suppose, are the ordinary warts that some children develop; these are caused by special types of viruses. Another form of wart develops from the epidermis in later life and as far as we know is not caused by a virus. These warty spots occur mainly on the trunk and face and increase in number as one ages—like barnacles on a rusting ship. They are known as seborrhoeic warts, and are usually slightly raised-up, light-brown growths with a rough surface. They are quite benign and usually don't cause symptoms. Sometimes they irritate or become infected or catch in clothes. It is important to distinguish these seborrhoeic warts from more aggressive skin growths.

Solar keratosis

One of the most frequently-encountered disorders resulting from being in the strong sun over many years is known as solar keratosis. This is not a cancer, but represents a pre-malignant disorder. The solar keratosis is usually small (less than 1 centimetre or half an inch in diameter), flat or slightly raised up above the skin surface, and its surface is often scaly or quite hard and

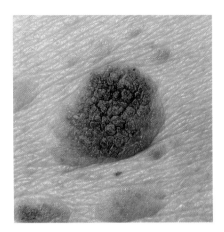

Typical common seborrhoeic wart.

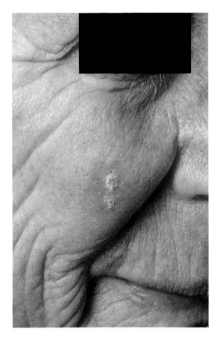

warty. Its colour is usually pink, but may be fawn or even brownish. Sometimes the surface is very heaped up and horn-like. These warty areas occur mainly in the sun-exposed parts of the skin, particularly the forehead, nose, tips of the ears, upper cheeks, the backs of the hands and the lower legs in women. Of course they may be seen elsewhere too, depending on which parts of the skin have been exposed over the years. They occur predominantly in fair-skinned individuals who have signs of chronic solar damage (see Chapter 4). Many of these spots may occur in the same patient; in fact there is some evidence that all the sun-exposed skin in these patients shows abnormalities similar to those observed in the solar keratosis, even

Pink, scaling patch on cheek due to solar keratosis.

though the skin doesn't show any obvious abnormality other than the effects of the sun.

Mostly, then, these solar keratoses are small warty or rough patches on visible sun-exposed areas of skin. They are annoying, unbeautiful little excrescences, but for the most part have no dire effect on their owner. Despite their potential for progression from unobtrusive static pre-malignant lesions to aggressive cancers, the transformation is really very uncommon. In fact, some actually seem to go away of their own accord. The proportion that become malignant is not known accurately but is certainly very small—my guess would be of the order of 0.1 to 0.2 per cent. It may be that the majority are kept in check by the body's own immune defence system, and this could also be the reason why some actually disappear—the immune system gets the upper hand and rejects the pre-malignant cells because they don't seem to be a normal part of the body.

Solar keratoses are extremely common in some parts of the world. For example, in some parts of Australia the population is at high risk from all types of injury from sun exposure and in one survey of one city it was found that just over half the population over the age of 40 had at least one solar keratosis. To put this figure in a European context, in a recent study in South Glamorgan we found that about 24 per cent of individuals over the age of 60 had at least one solar keratosis. As already mentioned, fair-skinned people are more prone to develop these 'sun-warts', as they are sometimes called, because of a deficiency of protective melanin in their skin (see Chapter 3). The populations of Scotland, Ireland and Wales seem particularly at risk of developing types of skin cancer. Of course the Celtic origins of the inhabitants of these areas have been much diluted over the years, but there are still many fair and red-haired Celtic types who are extremely sensitive to damage from the sun. Paradoxically, though, many Scots, Welsh and Irish individuals who are not all that fair also seem to be prone to the problem, and why this should be so is puzzling and of great interest.

If a solar keratosis does 'move on' and progress to a cancer, what are the signs? An early change is an increase in size of the 'rogue' keratosis. It also increases in thickness and may become inflamed and itchy. When this sort of cancer stays more or less like a large, thickened keratosis and doesn't break out of the confines of the epidermis it is known as an intra-epidermal epithelioma. This is also called Bowen's disease, after the dermatologist who originally described it. Areas of Bowen's disease can reach 1 to 2 inches (5–10 cm) in diameter if left untreated, and this surface skin often becomes quite red and scaly so that it is not uncommon for them to be misdiagnosed as patches of the common scaling disease psoriasis. Generally, this type of lesion (lesion is a general term meaning any localized abnormality of tissue) doesn't cause any real medical problem, although it may be unsightly.

If the abnormal cells of Bowen's disease break out from the epidermis and start to invade the dermis we have the sort of cancer known as a squamous cell carcinoma. This usually enlarges quite quickly to form a tumour or a large thickened patch. The surface may be hard and warty or may break down to form an ulcer. This type of cancer is potentially dangerous and needs treatment urgently before it spreads (see

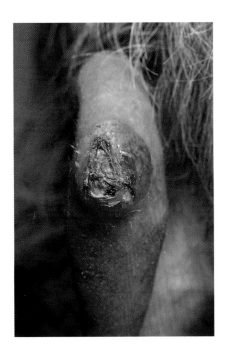

Large crusted nodule on the ear of an elderly man caused by squamous cell carcinoma.

genitals, but then this is not often due to sun exposure, and is outside the remit of this book!

There is one type of growth that occurs in the light-exposed areas of the skin that seems to heal spontaneously after reaching a particular size. This odd lesion is called a keratoacanthoma. It grows rapidly within 6 to 12 weeks and quite fittingly looks like a small volcano, with steep walls and a sort of crater at the top. After the period of growth it starts to wither away.

Rodent ulcers

This odd name is given to a very special sort of skin cancer that is more scientifically called a basal cell carcinoma. It is quite common, especially on fair-skinned individuals who have had quite a lot of sun exposure. Something like 4 to 6 per cent of all my new patients have a rodent ulcer. It is a very slow-growing form of cancer that gradually enlarges over the years and eventually ulcerates. The resulting ulcer is then said to resemble a rat bite, which is why our forebears gave this odd name to the disorder. Typically it causes a whitish or pinkish nodule to appear somewhere on the skin of the face. Actually it can occur anywhere on hair-bearing skin, but the great majority occur over the face. A few occur on the trunk and less occur on the limbs. Usually the spot very slowly infiltrates the tissues locally, and it never spreads to other parts of

pages 64-66). However, although potentially dangerous, it really is quite uncommon for anyone to come to any serious harm with them. This is because most cancers of this type grow very slowly and tend not to spread rapidly—only a few are really aggressive. When, as is rarely the case, the cancer does spread quickly, the malignant cells find their way into the lymph glands and if untreated can spread further, all over the body. When these growths affect the ear or the lip they tend to be more dangerous. The same is true if the cancer affects the

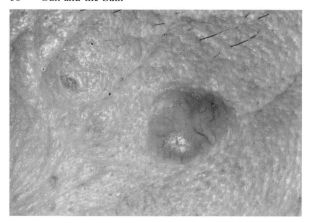

Nodule on skin of the face caused by basal cell carcinoma (rodent ulcer).

the body, or at least only extremely rarely.

A rodent ulcer can cause problems if left untreated as the local invasion of tissues it causes can be very destructive, but in general the outlook is excellent. Apart from the small nodule which is characteristic of a rodent ulcer, it may also take on the form of an ulcer or scaly patch. It can also be black, and then be confused with a malignant melanoma (see later). More rarely, it can look just like a scar.

Malignant melanoma—the 'black cancer'

This type of skin cancer has achieved a kind of grim reputation because of its ability to kill if left untreated.

There are few people in the UK who have not heard of moles changing their character and turning into cancer, and it is evident that they find this information frightening. It is important that the public are made more aware of the dangers as it is only by early diagnosis that we can hope to cure the disease, yet it seems difficult to educate without alarming. It is now commonplace to have one or more individuals in each of my clinics who are worried about one or other of their moles. Although the great majority of these worried individuals have simple benign moles, we do see some who have very early forms of malignant melanoma; however, because they have come to see us at an early stage, they can be completely cured.

What is this disease, then, that has stimulated so much discussion? Malignant melanoma is a cancer of the pigment-producing cells, the melanocytes. About half of these growths start in moles, while the other half start in previously unblemished skin. Moles are birthmarks which all white-skinned people possess. Birthmarks (a birthmark is sometimes known as a naevus) are odd areas of skin whose origins were present at birth, and in which there are benign growths of different kinds of tissue—blood vessels in 'strawberry marks', fatty tissue in some soft lumps, and the pigment-producing melanocytes in moles. White-skinned individuals have about a dozen or so moles on their skin on average, so there is no point in our becoming introspective about every wretched little brown spot that we can see on our skin. As most readers will be aware, moles are of an enormous variety of shapes, sizes and depths of pigmentation. Flat ones tend to be called lentigos and they have to be distinguished from freckles that aren't really birthmarks at all but areas of increased pigmentation that develop after stimulation by the sun's rays.

Some moles are very disfiguring as they cover quite large areas of the skin's surface. These tend to cover the area around the hips or around the shoulders and are known as 'bathing trunk' or 'cape' naevuses, respectively. They are rare, and congenital, i.e. they are there from birth. Smaller moles are also sometimes present at birth and tend to be larger and more irregular in shape than ordinary moles that develop in childhood. There seems to

be a slightly increased risk of developing a malignant melanoma in congenital moles, and the larger the mole, the greater the risk.

There are two other uncommon varieties of mole that also need comment from the standpoint of malignant melanoma. The first of these, the juvenile melanoma, is really only important from the professional's point of view but is of sufficient interest to mention here. The juvenile melanoma, not unexpectedly, occurs predominantly in children and young teenagers. The spots themselves certainly don't look like ordinary moles as they are often pink or red and have an odd sort of pitted or wrinkled surface. They tend to disappear spontaneously in early adult life. They are quite benign and harmless, but present a frightening picture down the microscope if they are removed, as they can look just like malignant melanoma.

The other condition that needs description has more significance. This is the so-called dysplastic mole syndrome in which there are many odd-looking moles occurring over the skin surface. This disorder, which has only been known about since the mid-1970s, is also known as the B-K mole syndrome, after the two families in which it was first found. One unusual feature of the dysplastic mole syndrome is that in some of the affected individuals it seems to run in families. The odd moles of the dysplastic mole syndrome are slightly more prominent than ordinary moles and more irregular in outline, and tend to be irregular

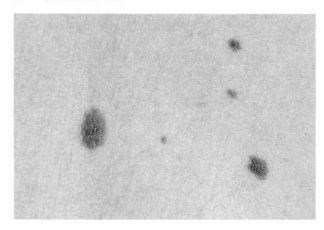

Several odd looking moles on the back of a young man who has dysplastic mole syndrome. These moles are more likely to become malignant than ordinary moles.

in the degree of pigmentation. The importance of this strange disorder is that there is an appreciably higher risk of the individual moles developing into a malignant melanoma, and the risk is greater if the condition runs in the family.

All moles seem to go through a life cycle in which they develop and grow before finally degenerating and disappearing. Because of this, old people's skin has many fewer moles than that of young adults because most of the moles have degenerated. Although the usual time for moles to start to develop is in childhood and early adolescence, they can make their debut later in life— in the 20s and 30s. This sometimes alarms people as they believe that the appearance of a new mole must mean that it is a cancer.

Another occurrence that quite often frightens people is the development of inflammation in a mole. The inflammation can be due to several different problems. The commonest reason for the mole to be inflamed is that one of the hairs in the mole has either been plucked or somehow the hair follicle has become twisted and has burst. When this is the cause the pain, tenderness, swelling and pinkness improve after a week or two, without any treatment. Another common cause for a mild type of inflammation is if the mole is being 'rejected' by the body. The rejection process results in a white halo developing around the mole and the mole itself gradually disappearing. During the rejection process the skin may become pink and slightly itchy.

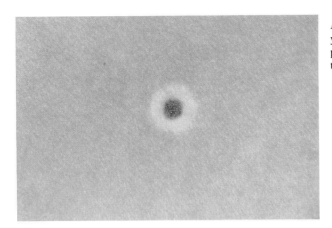

A halo naevus in a young man. The white patch had appeared in the previous 6 months.

Signs of malignancy

As I said before, the best way we have of improving the outlook for this form of cancer is early diagnosis. Everyone should know the danger signals. If someone becomes worried about one of their moles or any pigmented spot the best policy is to go straightaway to their general practitioner. In some hospitals there are walk-in clinics for patients who believe that they may have a malignant melanoma. These have the advantage of avoiding the delay of appointments, but in some specialists' view these clinics also have major disadvantages, so that they are not universally popular.

The major causes of delay in being treated are still lack of awareness of the significance of the changes taking place

and fear of finding out the diagnosis. It must also be said that it is really quite difficult for doctors to be certain about the diagnosis from just looking at a pigmented spot. Some lesions are quite easy to diagnose but some are not, and need to be examined under the microscope after being removed before one can be confident as to exactly what they are.

Enlargement of a pre-existing mole or the appearance of a new pigmented nodule or patch are important signs of the development of malignant melanoma. The speed with which the increase in size takes place is quite variable and obviously the more rapidly enlargement takes place the more worrisome is a particular lesion. Change in colour is also a major pointer to malignancy; increase in the pigmentation and

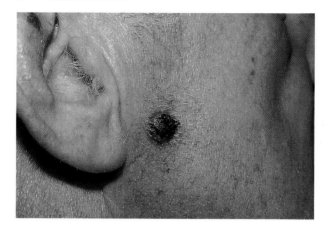

Malignant melanoma of the skin on the face of an elderly man. This lesion had enlarged over the previous 4 months and was becoming darker and more irregular.

irregularity of the degree of pigmentation across the lesion are both important signs. Furthermore, change in shape may signify the development of malignancy, as asymmetry and irregularity in outline are also signs of melanoma. Ulceration and bleeding are less common but equally strong signals that cancerous change may have taken place. Soreness and itchiness may also accompany the development of malignant melanoma. If these changes occur or you are concerned about the possibility, it is important that you seek a medical opinion as soon as possible.

These are actually several types of malignant melanoma. Some sorts tend to invade upwards towards the surface and then sideways. These are known as superficial spreading melanomas and have high cure rates and a good outlook. Others seem to have the ability to invade deeply and form nodules in the skin. These nodular melanomas have a worse outlook than the superficial sort and it has been found that the cure rate depends almost entirely on the depth to which the malignant tissue has invaded the skin. Another sort is really quite benign, even when compared to the superficial spreading sort. This type characteristically forms a flat area of pigmentation that mostly occurs on the face of elderly individuals. The patch is usually irregular and often has darker patches within it. This so-called malignant freckle gradually increases in size over many years, not causing anything other than slight cosmetic problems. However, in many cases a thickening eventually appears at one point in the freckle which then behaves just like the nodular malignant melanoma described above. A quite rare variety of malignant melanoma occurs around the fingernails or toenails or on the palms and soles. Curiously enough, this type (known as acral lentiginous melanoma), although rare in white-skinned subjects, is the commonest type of malignant melanoma in Asian and African peoples.

How common is it?

Malignant melanoma can occur at any age in adult life and, unlike most other forms of cancer, doesn't appear to be more frequent in older age groups. It is slightly more common in women. Overall it is an uncommon sort of disease in the UK, being responsible for one per cent of all cancers. However, there has been a startling increase in the frequency with which malignant melanoma occurs throughout the Western world, with a doubling of the frequency of the disease each decade since records started. Recently it has been computed that in Scotland there has been a 7 per cent increase in the incidence of malignant melanoma each year since 1972. In some parts of the world it is much more of a problem—notably in Australia, where it accounts for 7 per cent of all cancers in New South Wales and affects something like 4.5 people

per thousand per year in Queensland. It is also reported as being seen quite frequently in white populations in other sunny areas of the world, including Arizona, Hawaii and Israel. By the year 2000 there will be a 1 per cent lifetime risk of developing melanoma in the citizens of the United States. There seems to be a direct relationship between the distance one is from the equator and the likelihood of developing the disease.

One quite interesting fact about the disease is that not only does its occurrence seem to be related to the amount of UVR received but that it also frequently occurs on apparently unexposed areas of the trunk. It has been suggested that this is due to the sun causing a 'melanoma factor' to be released into the blood from the exposed areas. An alternative and more reasonable suggestion is that the unexposed sites may in fact be exposed in short sharp bursts during holidays and that acute sunburn may be hazardous in this respect. In support of this idea is the fact that melanoma appears to occur more commonly after good summers and, indeed, after increased sunspot activity (see Chapter 2)!

Outlook for patients with melanoma

The danger of melanoma is that it may spread while the lesion is still quite small. None the less, it must be strongly emphasized that if the area is removed while still confined to the superficial part of the skin the outlook is very good. Thus, while the overall survival rate for patients with all stages of the disease is approximately 80 per cent in the first five years after diagnosis and treatment, it is 100 per cent for very early and superficial lesions. When the disease is unfortunately allowed to spread it can do so both locally in the skin and, via the bloodstream, throughout the body. When spread does occur it is extremely unpredictable, and even when there are many metastatic tumours throughout the body the disease can suddenly and spontaneously start to improve and even ultimately disappear. In fact the outlook is directly related to the depth of invasion in the skin, and probably the most important indicator of the likelihood of survival, providing that the melanoma is confined to the skin, is the measurement down the microscope of the thickness of the melanoma after its removal.

To some extent the outlook depends on who you are and on which part of the body the melanoma occurs. Probably the best outlook is for a young or middle-aged woman with a melanoma on the trunk or arm and the worst is for a man with a melanoma on the back. These broad generalizations come from retrospective statistical analysis of the results in large numbers of patients, and of course it is impossible to be certain about the outlook in any one individual patient.

The diagnosis of skin cancer

Patients often turn up in our clinics expecting a confident diagnosis from a doctor after he or she has simply looked at the spot or mole in question.

I wish it was always that simple! In fact when the accuracy of our clinical judgment is put to the test we don't score as well as we think we should—even the most experienced and careful dermatologists get no more than about 75 per cent of the spots right. The pigmented spots are especially difficult, and it can be almost impossible to distinguish some moles from some melanomas. Brown or black 'old age' warts can also confuse the issue. Frequently the final decision is only made by a detailed microscopic examination of the spot after it has been removed, although it may well be that in the future we will have better techniques, with special instruments which can painlessly examine the spot on the skin using ultrasound or magnetic resonance imaging.

Ways of treating skin cancer

The treatment chosen for a patient with skin cancer will depend on which particular type of cancer has been diagnosed and what stage it has reached. It will also be influenced by the area of skin involved and the age, sex and general condition of the person affected, as well as the experience and preference of the doctor.

The large majority of skin cancers present no real problem. Most lesions of basal cell carcinoma, squamous cell carcinoma and even melanoma can be removed by simple surgery, usually under local anaesthetic, and the procedure is less troublesome (and less unpleasant!) than going to the dentist. Occasionally it is clear that surgical removal will require special skills and take a little longer than is reasonable for an ordinary outpatient procedure, and dermatologists with the necessary experience and training are asked for assistance. If the cancer has spread to involve nearby tissues, more extensive surgery and some grafting may be required. Occasionally a technique known as microsurgery is employed. In this procedure sections of the affected skin are cut away and checked microscopically to see whether they contain tumour. This process is repeated until it can be seen that all the affected skin has been removed. In cases of melanoma the surgeon hopes to remove all the cancerous cells by removing some of the normal-looking skin around the lesion as well.

Solar keratoses and patches of .Bowen's disease may be dealt with by ordinary surgical techniques or may be removed by some other locally-destructive method. Freezing the skin with liquid nitrogen, solid carbon dioxide or some other very cold substance is sometimes employed. The opposite but equally effective approach is to destroy the growth by some form of heat. Usually electrical cautery is employed, using an electrically-heated wire loop. Chemical destruction is also employed by some doctors, using a range of locally corrosive substances. A rather special adaptation of this technique, called Moh's chemosurgery after the surgeon who devised it, has been used by a few specially-trained doctors. This method, which is similar to the microsurgery described above, is also designed to deal with large growths that have deeply infiltrated the tissues of the face. The growth is first killed with a chemical agent and then removed surgically, allowing the surgeon to see just how much tissue needs to be removed.

Cancers of other organs are sometimes treated by drugs that are meant to kill off the cancer cells but leave the normal tissues untouched. Unfortunately these drugs are quite toxic, usually too toxic to be taken by mouth to treat small growths of the skin. However, one of these, called 5-fluorouracil, has been used very successfully in an ointment for the treatment of solar keratoses.

Another method sometimes used for destroying the growths is X-rays. X-rays are not used for skin cancer as much as they were at one time because of the disadvantages of the method, one particular disadvantage being that the dose of X-rays is divided so that several trips to the hospital are required for the full course of treatment. Another is that the affected area may show scarring or at least signs of where the radiation was directed on to the skin.

New drugs and methods of dealing with cancer are constantly being developed, and I will mention just a few of these here. Vitamin A-like drugs, known as retinoids (see also Chapter 5), seem to have both a protective effect and an anti-cancer action. Some of these drugs can be given by mouth while others can be used directly on the affected area. Acitretin, a retinoid used mainly for patients severely affected with the skin disease psoriasis or with congenital skin disorders, and isotretinoin, a retinoid used for severe acne, have both been used to treat patients with multiple skin cancers. The drugs seem to have helped many of these patients but are not suitable for all because of their side-effects. Tretinoin, another retinoid usually used in a cream or lotion in the treatment of acne, has also been used in the treatment of multiple solar keratoses with some success. It is likely that newer, more effective, retinoid drugs with fewer side-effects will be available in the not too distant future.

Another new exciting anti-cancer drug is based on one of the body's defence agents. This material, known as interferon, has to be administered by injection directly into the growths themselves on several occasions but seems to have been quite effective in some patients.

One of the most important aspects of treating patients with skin cancer is the prevention of further problems. It has to be recognized that if one growth occurs in a sun-exposed site then it is quite likely that another will pop up nearby sooner or later. Forewarned is forearmed, so that when and if a new lesion appears the patient can recognize the disorder for what it is and arrange to see the doctor as soon as possible. There is also some evidence that if sunscreens are used regularly and further damage to the skin is avoided there is somewhat less of a chance that further growths will develop.

The sun and skin cancer

When I see a patient who has a small growth on the skin that I believe has been caused by exposure to the sun over many years, as well as explaining what the condition is and what we intend to do about it, I also try to explain that the sun is mainly to blame. I think it quite important to do this to try to cut down on the chances of the patient developing any more similar growths. Mostly my explanations and suggestions are politely heard but received with some degree of scepticism. Interestingly, a recent survey in the United States found that, while half of the people asked knew about the relationship between sunbathing and skin cancer, very few seemed to act on the information; about one-third still actively tried to obtain a suntan and some 25 per cent took no precautions against the sun at all. I think this is rather sad but, being an optimist, I believe that public attitudes will gradually alter, and it is important to try to point out the dangers, even if they are not always instantaneously heeded.

The evidence that persistent exposure to the sun is a potent cause of skin cancer is overwhelming. The great majority of the common types of skin cancer occur on the face and the backs of the hands—those parts of the skin's surface that are consistently exposed to the sun. In bald-headed men it is quite common for growths to develop over the bald pate—no longer protected by the hair from solar radiation. Women also develop these disorders on the fronts of the lower legs, below the hemline. The back of the neck, the tops of the ears in men and the upper part of the front of the chest are also exposed sites and may develop the same kinds of skin cancer.

Another very important piece of evidence concerns the geography of skin cancer. I once worked in Miami and was astounded to see the large numbers of patients with one form or another of neoplastic disease of the skin. Since then I have also attended clinics in Texas and Australia, and it is evident to me that skin cancer in one form or another is very common in fair-skinned individuals who have lived out in the sun over long periods. Of course it is by no means solely my experience but the combined experience of many dermatologists over many years that makes it quite clear that the more sun exposure received

the greater the likelihood of developing skin cancer. There are good data to relate the occurrence of certain types of skin cancer in different places to the geographical latitude, and there can be little doubt that there is a strong relationship between the accumulated dose of solar irradiation received and the chance of skin cancer developing.

Two factors tend to obscure the relationship. The first is the degree of protective skin pigmentation. As I have mentioned many times already, fair-skinned individuals are much more vulnerable than darker folk. Clearly the frequency with which skin cancer occurs in a population will depend not only on the nearness to the equator and the average number of sunshine hours per day, but on the relative numbers of fair- and dark-skinned subjects. The other major factor hiding the relationship is that different types of skin cancer seem to have different kinds of relationships to the amount of solar energy received. Solar keratoses and squamous cell carcinoma seem to have a fairly simple relationship in that they virtually only occur on sun-exposed, and indeed severely sun-damaged, sites on the skin surface. It is not quite so simple for basal cell carcinoma or for malignant melanoma, as both sometimes occur in non-sun-exposed sites. In many of the cases in which basal cell carcinoma occurs in non-sun-exposed sites it seems that the occurrence of the growth is determined by genetic influences. Malignant melanoma has proved a major puzzle, but there is no doubting the considerable increased frequency of the disease in the hotter sunny areas of the world, despite the fact that it often occurs on parts of the body that are usually covered. It has been suggested that short intense episodes of sun exposure may predispose to melanoma, making the two-week Mediterranean skin-grilling type of holiday somewhat hazardous if no precautions are taken.

Apart from the observations just discussed, there have been many planned experiments which tend to confirm that the UVR in the sun's spectrum has a cancer-producing (carcinogenic) effect. Mostly the experiments have involved shining artifically-produced UVR on laboratory mice over periods of several weeks or months. Although their skin has only broad similarities to human skin, there is no doubt that the effects of this type of irradiation bear an uncanny resemblance to the effects of sun on human skin. Using this approach researchers have been able to incriminate UVB as the major waveband responsible for the carcinogenic effects of solar exposure (see Chapter 2). UVA—the long-wave portion of solar UVR—also has some carcinogenic effects, but because its intensity is comparatively low in sunshine it is probably much less important under ordinary circumstances. However, UVA does give rise to problems when it is used as a form of treatment for psoriasis (see Chapter 8).

What actually happens in cells and tissues to make them turn cancerous after they have been injured by UVR? We are a long way from knowing how many mechanisms are involved and all the various steps, but some interesting things have come to light. UVR seems to damage the cells' genetic material—its deoxyribonucleic acid, or DNA. Normally there are special enzymes in the nucleus of the cell which repair the UVR-induced damage. It is possible that under some circumstances the repair is incorrect or incomplete, allowing the cell to lose its genetic controls. In one unusual congenital disease called xeroderma pigmentosum there is a deficiency in one of the repair enzymes and skin cancers may develop early in life.

Another important effect of UVR may be on the skin's capacity to protect itself immunologically via the Langerhans cells (see Chapter 3). It may be that when rogue cancer cells develop they are normally destroyed by the immune defences if these are intact. If the immune defences are compromised by the action of UVR in depleting the skin of Langerhans cells, any cancer cells that emerge in the skin may be allowed to flourish. Patients who have had a kidney (or some other organ) transplanted into their bodies are maintained on special drugs known as immunosuppressive agents to prevent the body's immune defences from rejecting the new organ. The immunosuppression seems to have one unfortunate effect—it allows the development of many skin cancers. Up to 20 per cent of patients in the UK with transplanted kidneys may be affected with growths of the skin in this way within 10 years of the operation, and the figures are somewhat greater in sunnier countries. Patients with AIDS also have depressed immunity and have the tendency to develop some types of skin cancer.

As stated before, there can be no doubt that the sun is an important cause of skin cancer but it should not be imagined that it is the only cause. We know that some kinds of virus may be important, that some chemicals may also play a role, and that genetic influences are sometimes to blame. For example, it has been known for many years that skin cancer may be caused by radiation with X-rays, as the early X-ray doctors found out to their own cost. Heat injury may also cause skin cancer and very occasionally a growth is found on the front of the legs of poor elderly folk who have been trying to keep warm by sitting by the fire. Because of this, scientists have wondered whether the heating effect of the sun may contribute to the development of skin cancer, but although it may have a small effect it is not thought to be very important. Sometimes several of these factors combine to allow skin cancer to develop. None the less, the single most potent provocation, and the one responsible for by far the largest number of skin cancers, is the UVR from the sun.

7

Sunshine— the good side

Everyone loves to see the sun—that is, everyone in north-west Europe. Sailors in the Pacific Ocean or the Persian Gulf and farmers in the southern United States wouldn't mind the weather being cloudy once in a while. It is none the less true that in general the human species is gladdened by the sun and saddened by its being hidden by cloud, storm, night or eclipse.

There are obvious physical reasons why this should be so. The sun warms us and enables comfortable living without recourse to heavy clothes, shelter or fires. Although we are homeothermic creatures—that is, we are designed to keep our body temperature constant—it may be that it is less 'energy-expensive' on the part of our body chemistry to take advantage of external sources of heat. Certainly most vertebrate species of animals bask in the sun whenever the opportunity arises, unless they are in danger of overheating, in which case they beat a rapid retreat to the shade. The major danger for us in north-west Europe, though, is not overheating but underheating and the development of hypothermia in the

socially deprived and elderly population. Obviously heating from the sun has considerable importance for our bodies.

The heat supplied by the sun may have other benefits that are less well understood. For example, the healing of skin wounds may be hastened by increasing the surface temperature of the skin to the temperature of blood heat. Normally skin surface temperature is several degrees below that of blood; when heated directly by the sun its temperature rises and many sorts of chemical activity in the skin are stimulated, including the rate of epidermal cell migration and cell division, both of which are important in wound healing.

Light is the other major physical influence that the sun wields over our lives. Virtually all our light comes ultimately from the sun—even moonlight is sunlight reflected from the moon's surface. Our whole lives are geared to information obtained through the agency of sunlight or one of its substitutes. Information conveyed to us by our senses of hearing and touch are of course important, and indeed pre-eminent in a blind person, but of secondary importance in comparison with vision in those with normal sight. Sunlight and white light in fact are made up of all the colours of the rainbow. Something appears coloured because it absorbs some parts of this colour spectrum and reflects others (see Chapter 2). Pause for just a moment when you are next in a city centre. See the cars, the shop windows, the colourful goods on display in them, the posters and advertisements, and the 'variegate plumage' of the passers-by. All are testimony to the dominance of the visual and hence the central importance of light in our society. For the large majority of the population with normal sight the interplay of form, colour and texture provide important sources of pleasure in art forms, design and fashion. Many of us would feel deeply deprived without being able to feast our eyes on beautiful things once in a while. Throughout history mankind has demonstrated an innate need to create a visually appreciated expression of his emotions which is in harmony with his, and his peers', inherent view of the aesthetic. These activities are impossible without light.

As children we are frightened of the dark and associate the gloom with monsters, ghouls, ghosts and spirits. Even as adults all but the most stolid and steely (or perhaps the least imaginative) are unhappy in dark unlit alleys or the inky blackness of an unfamiliar house without light. The night is the time for crime and for doing all sorts of secretive forbidden things. Even when we have the technical ability to abolish the night with the mere flick of a switch and can flood the environment with light from neon tubes and other artificial sources, we retain a primitive fear of the dark.

'You are my sunshine, my only sunshine, you make me happy when skies are grey . . .'. The words of this popular old song say it all. In general, sunlight makes us happy: its absence and the dark makes us sad. The words that we use to describe mood are interesting in this context. 'She has a sunny disposition' usually signifies a bright, happy soul—there, quite unintentionally I've done it again, using the adjective 'bright' to describe a pleasant attribute rather than the intensity of light. 'He is in a black mood' means that the individual is in a foul temper or depressed, and if someone has a 'black soul' we think of them as being thoroughly evil.

Light does have a very important effect on mood. Think how miserable it can get in January or February during the long winter nights, when dark, overcast skies hang over the shortened days. Morale improves immediately the sun starts to shine, quite independently of the heating effect of the sun. Although the cheering uplifting effects of sunlight do not seem absolute, they are evident when contrasted to the effects of the absence of sunlight. For example, the people of southern Australia, or of any other sunny area, are roughly the same, temperamentally, as people anywhere else—they have much the same range of personalities and moods as any other population. However, their mood and outlook isn't nearly as much influenced by the sun as it is in those who live in the duller areas of the world, the morale-boosting effects of the sun being far more evident in countries that have long, dark and gloomy winters, as in Scandinavia.

To emphasize the profound effects that sunlight has on mood, there can be little more persuasive than the findings of recent research that there is a relationship between the number of suicides and the amount of clear sunshine at any particular latitude. Apparently it is the light that is important and not sunlight specifically. In support of this is the improvement after treatment with artificial light in patients with an odd psychiatric disease known as SAD (seasonal affective disorder). In this recently-described mental illness patients become pathologically depressed every winter and hypomanic in the summer time. In the treatment quite bright light has to be used—dim light won't do. Also, it's no good shining the light on the skin—it doesn't improve the patients; they have to see the light, but how the light stimulus is translated into mood changes is completely unknown.

The effects of sunshine are sufficiently marked and consistent to make one wonder if there isn't something more than just pleasure involved at seeing the sun but perhaps a physical effect on the endocrine glands of the body. For example, there is quite good evidence that light controls the reproductive cycles of some animals. Careful research has shown that this may be due to the effect of light on a secretion from a gland just at the front of the brain known as the pineal gland. This secretion is known as melatonin, and it seems to have quite interesting effects on the reproductive activity of small mammals, ensuring that the young are born in springtime. Whether there is some analogous

effect of light on reproductive activity in man is not clear. Perhaps there is something in the obsession that poets and romanticists have with the spring! It certainly can be shown that light affects the levels of melatonin in the human blood, but we just do not know what this means.

Vitamin D and rickets

Vitamin D is one of the fat-soluble vitamins found in all dairy products, including milk, butter, cheese, yoghurt and eggs. Vitamin D is also produced in the skin by the action of part of the sun's spectrum on a chemical rather like vitamin D (I will go into more detail about this later). Vitamin D is of vital importance in the development and growth of bones and their maintenance in a healthy state; in particular this vitamin is concerned with the way that calcium is made up into bones. If insufficient vitamin D is taken in the diet or produced in the skin, then problems start to develop in the bony skeleton. In children whose bones are developing, a deficiency of vitamin D causes softening and bowing of the bones and they do not grow normally. This tragic condition is known as rickets, and was once common in children of the impoverished populations of the industrial parts of Europe. This was because such people lived on an inadequate diet and because the smoke and grime in the atmosphere in these industrial regions prevented the sunlight from reaching the skin.

However, infants aren't the only age group whose bones may suffer because of a vitamin D deficiency. Softening, deformities and fractures can also occur in mature adults and the elderly. In recent years it has been recognized that some immigrants are particularly at risk. Asian women coming to the UK may be particularly in danger, partially because of an inadequate diet with insufficient vitamin D content but also because of their very limited exposure to the sun for cultural reasons.

It has also been found that the elderly are in real danger because of a vitamin D deficiency. Their bones are more vulnerable anyway, because of the ageing process, but to make matters worse their diet is often nutritionally poor and frequently deficient in vitamin D. If they are immobile and can't walk in the park or somehow get some sun exposure they will also have deficient vitamin D production in the skin. The consequence of all this is that their bones break when subjected to quite minor injuries. A frequent casualty is the thigh bone or femur. A fractured femur is always a serious affair and in the elderly it can be the final straw and ultimately the cause of death. So seriously is this taken now that it is being proposed that residents of homes for the elderly and of other types of long-stay accommodation should have regular sunbathing sessions with artificial sunlamps.

Interestingly, vitamin D itself is now thought to be quite important in the normal metabolism of many different types of cell as well as being vital to bone. It appears to be very much involved in the way that cells mature and grow, and recently vitamin D and similar compounds have been used successfully in creams and ointments to treat psoriasis.

Vitamin D production in the skin

Let us now return to the mechanism of vitamin D production in the skin. The story has gradually unfolded and become much clearer in recent years. It seems that there is a precursor chemical in the epidermis called 7-dehydrocholecalciferol. This is turned into pre-vitamin D after exposure to ultraviolet radiation in the UVB wavelength (see Chapter 2). This pre-vitamin D then changes to proper vitamin D under the influence of body heat and the action of enzymes in the kidneys. After the vitamin D has been produced it finds its way into the blood with the help of a special carrier protein, where it becomes involved in the metabolic control of the body's calcium balance.

It seems that relatively little exposure to the sun is sufficient for the manufacture of enough vitamin D to keep you healthy—one estimate suggested that walking around in normal light clothing for 30 to 60 minutes on a summer day would be enough to prevent vitamin D deficiency.

Solaria

The beneficial effect of sunshine was certainly recognized by our Victorian forebears. There was a solarium attached to many of the best seaside and spa hotels, as well as to the most lavish homes. The great glass-walled and -roofed rooms near the top of the building faced south to trap the afternoon sun. Whether there was any real benefit from these rather grand baroque structures is unknown; it seems most likely that their restfulness and acknowledged social exclusivity supplied the bulk of the benefit from their use.

Their use then spilled across into medical treatment, and exposure to the sun was a mainstay of the treatment of pulmonary tuberculosis. I remember the balconies attached to the tuberculosis wards of the older hospitals during my training. Some of these balconies were sheltered by glass, so that they looked like odd greenhouses perched on the sides of the otherwise grim hospital buildings. The mortality from pulmonary tuberculosis was frightful in those days, and the solarium treatment must have improved morale, if nothing else. There may have been some slight benefit in that the vitamin D produced by the sun's action on the skin did seem to have a small therapeutic effect.

Antimicrobial actions of UVR

Short-wave ultraviolet radiation, or UVC, is an effective antimicrobial agent. It has been used to 'disinfect' the surfaces of tough, solid articles—many of you must have seen the small cabinets flooded by a blue light used for sterilizing combs and brushes at some hairdressing salons. Short-wave UVR of this sort is lethal to all living cells, and life would not be possible on the earth's surface if all the UVC were not filtered out by the atmosphere (see Chapter 2). Even though no UVC reaches the earth's surface, the UVR that does reach the earth does seem to have some antimicrobial action. How it does this is not clear but it may be that the action of UVR on water and certain chemicals causes the production of hydrogen peroxide (a potent disinfectant) and other peroxides which then destroy the bacteria, fungi and viruses responsible for skin infections. The energy of UVR has many other photochemical effects on biological systems, including the denaturing of protein, and some of these may also be responsible for the antimicrobial action of UVR.

Recently another way in which UVR stimulates resistance to infection has come to light. Apparently the interaction of UVR with the skin results in the formation of an antifungal activity that is released into the blood, but the way this happens is unknown.

What role, if any, the sun has in regulating the normal population of bacteria and yeasts that we all carry on our skin surface is unknown. It may be true that scantily-dressed subjects in hot climates are less troubled by fungus infections or boils, but if this is the case there are many other explanations, aside from any effect of the sun. And it should also be noted that exposure to UVR *lowers* the skin's resistance by reducing the number of protective Langerhans cells in the epidermis (see page 19). These are the cells that start off an immunological attack against foreign invaders, and when they are reduced in large numbers the skin may be more vulnerable to infection.

Treatment of jaundice in the newborn

Some babies are jaundiced when born, especially those that are born prematurely. The jaundice is caused by a yellow pigment in the blood called bilirubin, which is present because their livers aren't mature enough to remove it in the usual fashion. When blue light of a wavelength slightly longer than that of UVA, i.e. about 440 nanometres, is shone on the babies for some hours, the amount of bilirubin in the blood decreases, and this treatment has been used for this type of neonatal jaundice for many years.

part it is the skin alone that absorbs any light or UVR energy that falls upon it.

Treatment of skin disorders using sunshine or artificial sources of ultraviolet light

In Chapter 7 I described some of the ways in which the sun's rays or artificial sunlight have in one form or another been used in medical treatments. Here I want to deal with some of the ways in which sunlight—UVR—or some other form of light have been used as medical treatments for skin disorders.

If you think about it, the skin is ideally placed for treatment with some form of light or UVR as, unlike with X-rays, tissues below the surface cannot take advantage of the therapeutic qualities of light rays—they are absorbed at or just below the skin surface. Long-wave UVR just penetrates to the superficial part of the dermis, and may irradiate some of the blood cells in the capillary blood vessels, but for the most

Tuberculosis of the skin

There is one special form of tuberculosis that is confined to the skin. It causes a great deal of inflammation, scarring and deformity, and is known as lupus vulgaris. Lupus is Latin for wolf and, as with lupus erythematosus, the disease has gained this curious name because of the supposed resemblance of the skin disorder to the bite of a wolf. The disorder was not uncommon in the poorer social classes and caused considerable cosmetic disability in those affected.

As with all forms of tuberculosis, prior to the development of streptomycin and other drugs in the 1950s there was little in the way of treatment. However, a Finnish dermatologist called Finsen had noticed that some patients with lupus vulgaris improved after being in the sun, and he set to work to find out why and, if possible, add to the chances of improvement. He constructed huge lamps where UVR was produced by carbon arcs. These Finsen lamps could concentrate their radiant energy on the skin and were found to yield moderately good results after a long course of treatment. Finsen was awarded a Nobel prize for this achievement. Interestingly the institute named after him in Copenhagen became a famous hospital for the treatment of skin disease and cancer, and remained open until 1987. Lupus vulgaris has now, luckily, become an extremely rare disorder, which anyway responds well to conventional antituberculosis drugs, making the Finsen lamp a redundant but historically interesting piece of equipment.

Psoriasis and its treatment by sun and UVR

Psoriasis is a common chronic scaling disorder of the skin that occurs in families and affects about 2 per cent of most populations surveyed. The red scaling patches usually only affect small areas, but sometimes nearly the whole body is involved. Quite a lot is known about the way the disease affects the skin, but its actual cause remains undiscovered, and in general its treatment is less than satisfactory. It was discovered many years ago that exposure to the sun seems to improve the disease. Many patients say that their red scaly patches tend to disappear quite spontaneously in the summertime after being out in the sun, but not all psoriatics are helped in this way, and some cases even seem to deteriorate after exposure to the sun.

UVR treatment

Ordinary sunlamps, which mostly emit rays in the sunburning UVB waveband, were used as a form of treatment for the disorder when I was in training, and are still used for some patients. Mostly patients had the treatment about three times per week until their rash improved, usually after some four to six weeks. The time of each exposure depended on the patient's tolerance and was designed to stop short of causing the redness of sunburn. It was found quite by chance that if lotions and ointments containing tar were used as well as the sunlamp treatment there was an even better chance of success, and this was the basis of inpatient treatment for severe psoriasis in many centres until quite recently. The tar seemed to have the effect of sensitizing the skin to the UVR in the sunlamp.

Another type of UVR treatment for psoriasis was developed in the early 1970s and is still in use. This is based on lamps that mainly emit their UVR in the non-sunburning long-wave UVA range. Such lamps have only been available in recent years and the tubes have to be specially constructed. By itself the UVA would not have much effect, but the skin is made sensitive to this waveband by giving a special photosensitizing psoralen drug beforehand (see page 35). Mostly the psoralen is 8-methoxypsoralen, and is usually given in tablet form about two hours before the patient is exposed to the UVA. The psoralen drug can also be given by painting it on the skin or by putting it into bathwater. The proper name for this form of treatment is photochemotherapy with UVA, but this is such a mouthful that it is

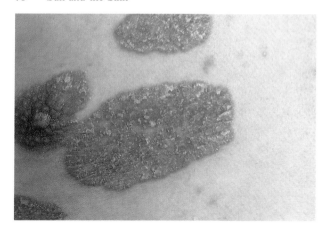

Typical plaques of psoriasis.

usually shortened to PUVA. Mostly the UVA is given in cabinets lined by special fluorescent lamps emitting exactly the right wavelength of ultraviolet radiation. Other ways of giving the UVA include canopies of lamps suspended over special beds, and smaller lamps for treating only the hands and feet or the scalp. The amount of UVA given is very carefully monitored because, as we shall see a little later, there are potential problems with this form of treatment.

In general, PUVA treatment is quite popular with patients because it is clean and there are no messy ointments to use. It makes you very tanned without the expense of going to the Mediterranean. And, of course, it works. It is effective in about 85 per cent of patients after about six weeks of treatment, and most don't seem to mind going about three times per week to the hospital or clinic where the PUVA treatment is based.

Recently PUVA has been given in combination with retinoid (vitamin-A-like) drugs in the treatment of psoriasis. This combination form of treatment rejoices in the acronym of RePUVA, and it seems even more effective than either treatment alone, and cuts down the dosage of both.

Side-effects from PUVA treatment are quite few, although if the treatment is not given with care it is possible for the patient to be quite severely burnt. The more worrying part about the treatment is its effects in the longer term. As explained elsewhere in this book, UVA has similar damaging effects as that part of the spectrum responsible for sunburn, and when artificially large amounts of UVA are administered then one can expect those effects to become evident. Wrinkling and other alterations due to solar elastosis (see Chapter 5) are evident in a proportion of patients treated with PUVA. These clinical signs are common in the community anyway, and the changes due to PUVA don't become evident until some time after the treatment has been started. Anyway, PUVA is not generally given to younger psoriatics, so that, all in all, these signs of premature ageing are not a major problem.

More disturbing is the appearance of small skin cancers. There has been quite a lot of discussion about the size of this risk. Researchers in the United States have reported that there may be up to 12 times the risk of developing a squamous cell carcinoma or a basal cell carcinoma some 10 years after treatment. However, European researchers from Vienna and Kiel do not agree, and have found that the increased risk was evident only in psoriatic patients who had had other forms of treatment in the past, particularly arsenic. The niceties of this debate aside, there is no-one who denies that PUVA can act as a stimulus to skin cancer; it just depends on the sensitivity of your skin and the dose received.

Many dermatologists are loath to start PUVA in fair-skinned patients under the age of 40 for just these reasons. There must also be an increased risk of skin cancer in patients who have tar and ordinary sunlamp treatment, but it does not appear to be as great as with PUVA. Patients being treated

with PUVA wear sunglasses that don't allow any UVA to reach the eyes, because there is an increased risk of cataracts, and they have to wear their sunglasses for the whole 24 hours after taking their tablets, because the sun's UVA can also stimulate the formation of cataracts while there is still some psoralen in the system.

Before leaving the subject of PUVA treatment for psoriasis, it ought to be said that all treatments have some inherent risk. Psoriasis can be a most disabling and unpleasant disorder, and PUVA has made life tolerable for many patients, so that as long as the individual patient fully understands the situation, the risk is probably justified.

Sun and psoriasis

As I mentioned at the beginning of this section, ordinary sunshine is well known to help clear psoriasis, and some sunny resorts have gone out of their way to attract psoriatic patients to their cities. The most famous of these is the Dead Sea resort in Israel, and the results obtained by the medical team who work there seem as good as for a comparable period of conventional inpatient treatment. It doesn't take much imagination to believe that this way of improving your skin problem is much more fun than going into hospital. Interestingly enough, for a 'package deal' of return flight, accommodation and treatment the cost is somewhat less than the cost to the

National Health Service for a comparable period in a British hospital!

But why is the Dead Sea treatment effective? It is claimed that bathing in the Dead Sea is itself helpful because of the salts and other materials in it, but there is really no evidence to support this. The Dead Sea is the lowest place on earth (it is 400 metres below sea level) and it is claimed that the thicker blanket of air between you and the sun filters out much of the sunburn UVB, allowing more of the UVA to fall on the skin in comparison with sites at sea level. Whether it is this greater dose of UVA or the bathing in the curious waters of the Dead Sea that has more effect, there is no doubt about the beauty and sense of calm about the place, and my guess is that this must also play some part in the therapy. Other resorts such as those by the Black Sea have also claimed that psoriatics benefit by a visit, but less is known about their results.

How the treatments work

And how does UVR work in psoriasis? Part of the answer lies in the damaging effect that UVR has on the epidermis (see page 18), which is very thickened and very active in psoriasis. UVR also damps down some of the immune processes in the skin (see pages 68 and 69) and this may also be helpful in this disease. There seems to be no difference between ordinary sunshine, Dead Sea sunshine, 'ordinary' artificial UVR

or PUVA when it comes to the nature of the anti-psoriatic effect on the skin.

Treatment of acne by UVR

Most of us have had acne during adolescence and early adult life. Mostly there are only a few slightly embarrassing teenage spots, but for some unlucky youngsters it is a dreadful persistent and deforming disease. As with

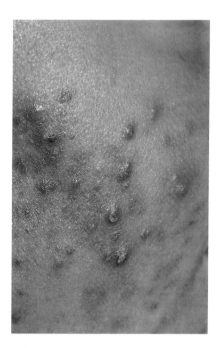

Inflamed spots in a young man with extensive acne.

psoriasis, many of those affected say that it improves in the summertime and after they have been out in the sun. Occasionally courses of treatment with UVR lamps are prescribed by dermatologists but, compared to its effects in psoriasis, UVR treatment is less useful and on the whole less frequently suggested, while PUVA seems to have no place in the treatment of acne.

However, one way in which UVR may improve acne is by helping to unplug the blocked hair follicles which are thought to play an important part in the events that lead to the development of acne spots. The UVR may also have an effect on the bacteria on the skin surface and in the hair follicles and on the inflammation in the skin, and both of these could be of some importance in helping to clear acne.

PUVA treatment for other skin disorders

PUVA can be a quite dramatic form of treatment for psoriasis and, as with any other effective and occasionally dramatic treatment, it has been tried in other skin disorders. Patients with bad generalized eczema may occasionally be helped, but this is not typical.

One disorder that does appear to be helped by PUVA is an uncommon form of skin cancer called mycosis fungoides. In this very slowly progressive disease, large red thick scaly patches develop over the skin surface, and PUVA treatment certainly does seem to hold it in check, at least in the early stage. The action of PUVA in this disease is extremely interesting and may be concerned with the action of UVR on a particular type of abnormal blood cell that seems at fault in this disease.

Some other uses of UVR

UVR in one form or another has been used in patients who, paradoxically, are oversensitive to it (see Chapter 4)! This is in the hope that with small controlled doses, which are increased on a regular basis, they may become more tolerant of ordinary UVR in the sun. This seems to be effective in some patients, but the treatment is extremely inconvenient and the individual runs the risk of developing the full-blown rash which he or she is trying to prevent.

UVR and light of various types have also been used to stimulate healing in ulcers and wounds that are slow to heal. Specifically, there has been a vogue for the use of one type of polarized yellow light in the treatment of chronic ulcers of the leg, but if and how this really works is something we will have to wait to see. Mention should also be made of a form of treatment for skin cancer that is at the moment experimental but will in the near future come into general use. This is photodynamic therapy, where light of different kinds is shone on tissues treated with a photosensitizing chemical of the porphyrin type. Early results are very promising and there is also hope that other diseases such as psoriasis may be treatable in this way.

Lasers

Before finishing this chapter something ought to be said about the medical use of lasers. Essentially lasers are very strong sources of monochromatic light, in which all the light energy is in the same phase. Because the energy doesn't spread out as with ordinary light, laser beams have a small band width and intense energy. For the most part they are useful for their destructive power, which can be quite finely controlled. Lasers can be constructed to emit beams at different wavelengths, whether in different devices (e.g. a ruby laser, emitting red light) or in the same device (a tunable laser). The particular dermatological application will require a particular type of laser. Lasers are best known for their use in the treatment of deforming red birthmarks or the removal of tattoos. They are also useful in the treatment of other types of skin tumour and even massive and deforming moles. More and more applications are being found for their use and it is my guess that this trend will continue.

9

Protection against the sun

We have moved on a bit from the times when the pith helmet or the French legionnaire's *kepi* were regarded as the be-all and end-all of protection against the sun. Information concerning the dangers of sun exposure has stimulated the development of sunscreeens and other types of protective agent, and there are now so many products available from doctors and over the counter that some type of guidance on how to choose them is required. Despite their profusion there is room for improvement, and the best advice to a patient who is very sensitive to UVR is still to limit the opportunities for actual exposure of the skin to the sun's rays.

Stay in the shade

Advice to stay indoors is not generally accepted with gratitude, but it is none the less the most useful advice that can be proferred to a patient who is extremely sensitive to UVR. However, although this is generally true, there are some qualifications.

Most rooms have windows, and window glass can let through some UVR. Most of the sunburn rays are cut out by ordinary window glass but it does let through long-wave UVA-type irradiation. As we learnt in Chapter 4, there are some conditions where UVA is the part of the UVR spectrum to be avoided and obviously patients who are sensitive just have to keep away from the windows as well.

Some unfortunate souls are also sensitive to some parts of the visible spectrum, and if they wish to stay rash-free they have no choice but to live in the dark, or at least in light of the colour to which they are not sensitive, until their sensitivity has passed. Even artificial light isn't completely safe. Ordinary tungsten-filament bulbs seem quite blameless, but neon tubes do emit some UVR which could be provocative to someone who is very sensitive. It is worth noting that UVR from the neon lights of offices and factories has been accused by a few researchers of contributing to the skin cancer problem.

Most people I know don't want to stay indoors all the time and need advice as to how to avoid or reduce damage from the sun when they do go outside. Obviously avoidance of the period of the most intense radiation from the sun is the most sensible. This means avoiding being out in the sun from 11.30 am to 2.30 pm, or at least taking special precautions during this time.

And what protection can the shade give? Well, oddly enough, not a great deal. Diffused light through the branches of a tree and reflected light from buildings, sea, sand or snow nearby may permit an unacceptable amount of UVR to reach the skin. Obviously, sitting under an umbrella on a beach is better than no protection, but it should not be imagined that this is adequate to prevent either short- or long-term damage.

Do clothes protect?

'Does clothing protect against solar damage?' is a frequently asked question. As with so many questions, the answer is, 'It depends'. It depends on the intensity of the sun and the length of exposure, as well as the type of clothing worn. It is easy to get a little sunburnt under a thin cotton blouse or shirt when walking on the beach at midday in the summer, and really intense sun may penetrate several layers of thin summer clothing. Remember, too, that tiny holes and gaps in clothing provide gateways for the sun, and the skin beneath may easily get burnt which can result in some very odd patterns of sunburn or rash, as on the feet of one sun-sensitive patient who had perforated leather shoes.

Hats can be very important to give some protection, not to stop our brains from overheating, as was once thought, but to prevent severe sunburn of the balding scalp in mature men—such as the author's. A broad-brimmed hat can also give some protection to the face, though wearing a Stetson-style cowboy hat may not be everyone's choice.

Sunscreens

So far we have briefly discussed avoidance, shade and clothing as ways of obtaining protection from the sun, and this is all that was available until the development of sunscreens. These go by different names, including sun creams, sun barriers and sun blocks. Their basic aim is to prevent the sun's rays from contacting the skin, and they are of two main types. The oldest type just produces a physical barrier to the sun—this method is simple and efficient but, in general, not cosmetically acceptable (see page 87). The other sort, which is becoming more sophisticated every year, contains different chemical agents that absorb the damaging parts of the sun's spectrum.

One term in particular needs explaining—the sun protection factor or SPF. This is meant to indicate the minimum time required for you to obtain a burn with the cream, compared to the minimum time required for a burn without the cream. So if it would take six minutes for you just to develop a persistent redness where the skin is exposed without a cream and, say 48 minutes with the cream, then the SPF of the cream would be 8.

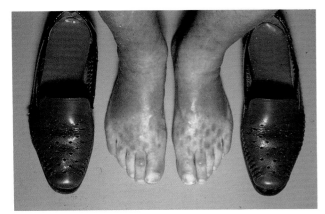

This elderly man developed an odd pattern of photosensitivity. The spotty pattern of rash on his feet was due to the holes in his shoes.

The higher the SPF, the more protective the cream. Fair-skinned individuals who are travelling to a very sunny area need creams with SPFs in excess of 15 to be sure of not burning.

Unfortunately, the subject is a little more complex than may at first appear, as SPF values are obtained experimentally using artificial sunlamps, for practical reasons. Unless the lamp has exactly the same spectrum as the sun, then it is difficult to be certain that the SPF of the preparation will be the same in the sun as when using the artificial UVR lamp. Some UVR lamps have what is known as a discontinuous spectrum, with radiation being strong at particular wavelengths (see Chapter 2). Others have a continuous spectrum similar to that of the sun, and are known as solar simulators. The authorities in the United States favour SPFs obtained using the solar simulator type of lamp, but those in Germany accept SPFs obtained using other artificial sources of UVR. The SPFs may therefore differ slightly, depending on which test system is used and the UVR-absorption characteristics of the particular cream in question.

Sun-barrier preparations need to have several properties, apart from the ability to filter out solar UVR. They need to be completely safe and not cause any rash or any other type of unwanted side-effect. In addition to being safe and effective at absorbing the UVR, they also have to stick on to the skin for longish periods and have to resist being washed off during swimming; after all, sunscreens are mostly used on the beach, and they are much more likely to prevent solar damage if they stay on the skin surface rather than having to be reapplied after every quick dip. In fact some of the protective compounds of some sunscreens actually seem to sink into the top part of the stratum corneum so that theoretically they ought to stay where they are put for quite long periods. Sunscreens must also be aesthetically acceptable; they have to smell, feel and look good, or they just won't be used.

Sunscreens have been much more efficient at reducing the threat from UVB than in cutting down the long-wave UVR. The reason for this is that chemical agents which absorb the sunburn UVB rays and which are suitable for use in a sunscreen preparation are more abundant than compounds that absorb UVA radiation. And in any case, it has always seemed more sensible to concentrate on screening out those rays that we know cause burning. However, in recent years it has been discovered that despite the weak 'burning' properties of the long-wave component of UVR, this segment of the solar spectrum does have quite marked damaging effects on the skin. We have already learnt (in Chapter 4) that many photosensitivity disorders of the skin are set off by UVA. Obviously patients with these disorders would appreciate a sunscreen that shielded them from the offending part of the spectrum and allowed them to go outdoors cautiously. Apart from any involvement in photosensitivities, it now seems that UVA may contribute to both photodamage and the development of skin cancer. The extent of the contribution is not clear, but it

seems quite likely that it is only a small part proportionately because of the relatively low biological effectiveness of UVA in other situations.

The fact that there are many sunscreens that screen out the burning rays of the sun but still allow some of the potentially damaging rays through has been somewhat alarming to some of us, as these screens remove the body's warning signals of redness and discomfort. There are some preparations that state that they are both UVA and UVB blockers, but in general the SPF that they quote applies only to their UVB protection and not to their ability to protect against UVA; in fact it is often the case that they have a relatively low protective effect against UVA. Various methods of determining the UVA protection of a sunscreen have been tried but none are entirely satisfactory. One method depends on the 'immediate pigment darkening effect' of UVA and how the sunscreen protects against this effect in volunteer subjects. Another is a laboratory test on the sunscreen which measures the transmission of UVA rays when the product is placed on a transparent tape. A 'star system' has been used to grade sunscreens, where the number of stars allotted to a particular preparation depends on the ratio of the SPF (protectivity against UVB) to protection offered against UVA.

The commonly used chemical screening agents which absorb radiation include *para*-aminobenzoic acid and its ester derivatives (such as padimate), anthranilates, cinnamates, benzophenones, and the camphor derivatives. (I have included the chemical names of the groups of compounds used so that you can recognize them on the tube or bottle!)

As mentioned at the beginning of this section, there are some preparations which just physically block out the rays. One of these, which was used to protect soldiers in World War II, was based on a veterinary petroleum jelly preparation and was known as 'red vet pet' for short. It was horrible to use, but extremely efficient. Creams and ointments containing zinc oxide, calamine, titanium dioxide, magnesium silicate and iron oxide can also be used for this purpose and are slightly more acceptable than 'red vet pet'! In fact any slightly opaque cream or ointment will have some protective effect.

The most important points about sunscreens are, firstly, to choose the best one for you and, secondly, to use the chosen product properly. A cream bought for when you are sitting on a Cornish beach for a couple of hours on a damp August afternoon just won't be suitable if you are windsurfing all day in the Mediterranean on a scorcher in July. Not only should the sunscreen fit the bill for the needed protection, but it should also be pleasing to use—or else it won't be used. A colourful tube may look splendid resting on a beach towel beside the transistor and the glass of Sangria, but to be of any use it has to be put over all the exposed skin. Depending on the particular preparation, it will then have to be re-applied every couple of hours or maybe after every swim.

Now that there have been campaigns on the radio and television about the dangers of sun exposure leading to skin cancer, it won't be long before the manufacturers claim that use of their product will prevent any such problem. Could there be any truth to this suggestion? Hard evidence in its support is very difficult to obtain, but there is some, and in my view it seems reasonable enough to make such a claim, providing that the preparations used are efficient absorbers of UVR. One group of scientists from Boston has recently computed that if sunscreens with an SPF of at least 15 were used regularly up to the age of 18 there would be a 78 per cent reduction in the likelihood of developing non-melanoma skin cancer.

Tan accelerators

There are several products on the market which claim to increase the degree of tanning as well as protect against burning. At one time there were preparations sold in the UK that contained a psoralen (5-methoxy-psoralen, or bergapten) which is a photosensitizing agent. The formulation also contained a UVB-absorbing chemical, and the idea of the material was both to protect against the UVB burning rays and to promote tanning by the combined action of UVA and the photosensitizing psoralen. Although there is no doubt that psoralen photosensitization can produce pigmentation, in practical terms there did not appear to be any real increased tanning when the product was used. Products containing 5-methoxypsoralen for this purpose are no longer available in the UK because of the possibility that they may accelerate UVA-induced damage, as well as tanning, and could even promote the development of skin cancer. However, they are still being sold elsewhere.

Another sort of 'tan accelerator' was promoted in the 1980s. To explain the basis of this type of accelerator we need to know a little about the chemical process of pigment production in the skin. Melanin, the brown-black pigment responsible for the 'tan', is produced by the pigment cells in the skin—the melanocytes. Melanin is a sort of protein made up of one amino acid in particular, called tyrosine (proteins are built up from amino acid 'building blocks'). The synthesis of melanin from tyrosine is promoted and accelerated by a copper-containing enzyme called tyrosinase, found within the melanocytes. The new tan accelerators attempt to stimulate this system, mostly by providing more tyrosine or mixtures containing tyrosine and other amino acids.

Despite the apparently scientific basis for these preparations, there is very little evidence that they do what they say they do. In fact one carefully-performed study into the effectiveness of one such product could find no special tanning properties whatsoever. To be effective the tyrosine in the tan accelerator has to penetrate the skin. In addition it has to come in contact with the tyrosinase enzyme, which in turn should not be fully occupied with the skin's own tyrosine that it normally makes into melanin. On both counts it seems that putting tyrosine on the skin and expecting an increase in the degree of melanin pigmentation is a forlorn hope, although this does not mean that it may not be possible to utilize this kind of approach with other substances in the future.

Brownish stains and tinted clinging cosmetic preparations are another sort of 'artificial tan'. Strictly speaking they are *not* tan accelerators but 'tan simulators', but they are widely used and it is worth pointing out the difference.

10

The future

Our attitude to 'fun in the sun' and suntanning are quite perceptibly changing, and the idea that being in the sun can be damaging is gradually getting home in the UK. The inclusion of 'a reduction in the incidence of skin cancer' in the Government's list of health gain objectives has certainly helped to promote the message in no small way. The increasing number of television and radio programmes, the newspaper interviews and magazine articles seem to be making some sort of impact. Perhaps ex-President Reagan's well-publicized skin cancers reinforced the message. Certainly the number of individuals who present to their general practitioner with a skin problem that they think may be a skin cancer or due to the sun has increased dramatically since the mid-1980s. The Australians and North Americans have been subjected to public health campaigns about the dangers of the sun over the past three decades. These seem to have made precious little difference to the amount of skin cancer in these communities so far, but I would guess that attitudes will change gradually. If one looks at the example of the campaigns against cigarette smoking, it is quite clear that even with intense efforts at public education there is only a limited response in the short term; beyond that intense effort there are diminishing returns.

The problems are of course much more important numerically in Australia and in the United States, and I am not surprised at the vigour and candour of the promotional pamphlets and booklets that I have seen from these countries. In the United States an institution has been set up, known as the Skin Cancer Foundation, whose specific aim is to promote research into the prevention and treatment of skin cancer. The American Academy of Dermatology has also been successful in lobbying for National Skin Cancer Detection Weeks, during which detection teams tour shopping centres and public places offering free examinations and advice. I believe that some such effort would be quite useful in the UK, but it has to be remembered that there are differences of scale and social organization between ourselves and the United States. There are about 7000 dermatologists in the United States to deal with a population of about 235 million, while we in the UK have about 270 dermatologists for a population of about 56 million. Given such statistics it is perhaps quite remarkable that current awareness in the public is at the level that it is.

Technical developments

It seems likely that much more efficient sunscreens will be developed in the future. Every year sees new compounds with more useful absorptive properties, and I would guess that in the next 10 years there will be sunscreens that can protect efficiently against the whole range of UVR. Whether they will be used by the public or not is another issue.

There are already some drugs which are taken by mouth that give some protection against UVR. I will be surprised if this avenue is not extensively explored by the pharmaceutical industry and perhaps exploited if successful. Think how much more convenient this would be than smearing yourself with some unpleasant greasy gunk before going into the sun!

You may remember that in Chapter 6 we discussed the damaging effect of UVR on the body's genetic material—deoxyribonucleic acid (DNA). There are intrinsic repair mechanisms that try to cobble together the broken strands of DNA after sun exposure. These mechanisms sometimes appear to be inherently weak or compromised in some way, and it is conceivable that a drug may be found to seek out the damaged DNA and give assistance in its repair. This could work in a similar way to the 'morning after' contraceptive pill—in other words, the tablet or pill would be taken *after* the sun damage had been sustained.

Recent work also suggests that the sun-damaged dermis—the part of the skin affected in wrinkling and in all the other signs of sun-induced skin ageing—can be stimulated to repair itself. As already mentioned in Chapter 5, the retinoid group of drugs have been shown to be active in just this way. The retinoid drugs may also be useful in preventing the development of skin cancer due to chronic damage from the sun. They certainly seem to have quite a good anti-cancer effect, and there are also signs that developments in these drugs could lead to safe compounds that could be given to actually prevent cancer.

Of course it is likely that there will be other developments on the drug treatment front, and we can look forward to a whole range of new treatments and preventive approaches in the next 10 to 20 years. Apart from chemical developments, however, it is also possible that there will be new techniques and new instruments that will allow diagnoses to be made early on, without sampling the skin by surgical methods. Ultrasound methods and magnetic resonance imaging techniques look quite promising on this front. It is also possible that further developments of lasers will enable us to treat forms of skin cancer more easily.

Despite the importance and the likelihood of all these pharmaceutical and technological developments in the next few years, they are comparatively unimportant beside one change that is quite slow in getting going—a change in attitude to sun exposure. As pointed out, we are making a start in this direction, but it needs sustaining and considerable encouragement.

Useful addresses

British Association of Dermatologists
3 St Andrew's Place
London NW1 4LB
Tel: 0171 935 8576

Cancer Information Service
3 Bath Place
London EC2A 3JR
Tel: 0171 613 2121

Cancer Research Campaign
6–10 Cambridge Terrace
London NW1 4JL
Tel: 0171 224 1333

D.E.B.R.A. (Dystrophic Epidermolysis
Bullosa Research Association)
D.E.B.R.A. House
13 Wellington Business Park
Duke's Ride
Crowthorne
Berkshire RG11 6LS
Tel: 01344 771961

Imperial Cancer Research Fund
44 Lincolns Inn Fields
London WC2A 3PX
Tel: 0171 242 0200

Lupus Group
Olivier Hanscombe
18 Stephenson Way
London NW1 2HD
Tel: 0171 916 1500

M.A.R.C.S. (Melanoma and Related
Cancers of the Skin) Resource Centre
Dermatology Treatment Centre
Level 3
Salisbury District Hospital
Salisbury
Wiltshire
Tel: 01722 415071

National Eczema Society
163 Eversholt Street
London NW1 1HT
Tel: 0171 388 4097

National Radiological Protection Board
Chilton
Didcot
Oxfordshire OX11 0RQ
Tel: 01235 831500

Psoriasis Association
7 Milton Street
Northampton NN2 7JG
Tel: 01604 711129

S.C.A.R. (Skin Charity to Advance
Research)
Department of Medicine
(Dermatology)
University of Wales College of
Medicine
Heath Park
Cardiff CF4 4XN
Tel: 01222 747747

The Skin Disease Research Fund
5 Lisle Street
London WC2H 7BJ

Index